Acid-Base and Electrolyte Handbook for Veterinary Technicians

Acid-Base and Electrolyte Handbook for Veterinary Technicians

EDITED BY

Angela Randels-Thorp

Team Director
1st Pet Veterinary Centers
Arizona

David Liss

Program Director-Veterinary Technology
Platt College
Los Angeles

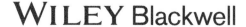

This edition first published 2017 © 2017 by John Wiley & Sons, Inc

Editorial Offices
1606 Golden Aspen Drive, Suites 103 and 104, Ames, Iowa 50010, USA
The Atrium, Southern Gate, Chichester, West Sussex, PO19 8SQ, UK
9600 Garsington Road, Oxford, OX4 2DQ, UK

For details of our global editorial offices, for customer services and for information about how to apply for permission to reuse the copyright material in this book please see our website at www.wiley.com/wiley-blackwell.

Library of Congress Cataloging-in-Publication Data

Names: Randels-Thorp, Angela, 1971– editor. | Liss, David, 1985– editor.
Title: Acid-base and electrolyte handbook for veterinary technicians / edited by
    Angela Randels-Thorp, David Liss.
Description: Ames, Iowa : John Wiley & Sons Inc., 2017. | Includes bibliographical references and index.
Identifiers: LCCN 2016035702| ISBN 9781118646540 (pbk.) | ISBN 9781118922880 (Adobe PDF)
Subjects: LCSH: Veterinary pathophysiology. | Acid-base imbalances. | Water-electrolyte imbalances. |
    MESH: Acid-Base Imbalance–veterinary | Acid-Base Equilibrium | Water-Electrolyte
    Imbalance–veterinary | Water-Electrolyte Balance | Animal Technicians
Classification: LCC SF910.W38 A25 2017 | NLM SF 910.W38 | DDC 636.089/607–dc23
LC record available at https://lccn.loc.gov/2016035702

A catalogue record for this book is available from the British Library.

Wiley also publishes its books in a variety of electronic formats. Some content that appears in print may not be available in electronic books.

Set in 9.5/13pt Meridien by SPi Global, Pondicherry, India

1   2017

Contents

List of Contributors, vii

Foreword – *Stephen P. DiBartola*, viii

About the Companion Website, x

1 Introduction to Acid-Base and Electrolytes, 1
Angela Randels-Thorp, CVT, VTS (ECC, SAIM) and David Liss,
RVT, VTS (ECC, SAIM)

2 Disorders of Sodium, 13
Angela Chapman, BSc (Hons), RVN, Dip HE CVN, Dip AVN, VTS (ECC)

3 Disorders of Chloride, 34
Meri Hall, RVT, LVT, CVT, LATG, VTS (SAIM)

4 Disorders of Potassium, 44
Dave Cowan, BA, CVT, VTS (ECC)

5 Disorders of Magnesium, 57
Louise O'Dwyer, MBA, BSc (Hons), VTS (Anaesthesia & ECC),
DipAVN (Medical & Surgical), RVN

6 Disorders of Phosphorus, 66
Louise O'Dwyer, MBA BSc (Hons), VTS (Anaesthesia & ECC), DipAVN
(Medical & Surgical), RVN

7 Disorders of Calcium, 79
Katherine Howie, RVN, VTS (ECC)

8 Traditional Acid-Base Physiology and Approach to Blood Gas, 102
Jo Woodison, RVT and Angela Randels-Thorp, CVT, VTS (ECC, SAIM)

9 Metabolic Blood Gas Disorders, 121
Eric Zamora-Moran, MBA, RVT, VTS (Anesthesia & Analgesia)

10 Respiratory Acid-Base Disorders, 136
Paula Plummer, LVT, VTS (ECC, SAIM)

11 Mixed Acid-Base Disorders, 152
Brandee Bean, CVT, VTS (ECC)

12   Strong Ion Approach to Acid-Base, 163
Angela Randels-Thorp, CVT, VTS (ECC, SAIM)

13   Companion Exotic Animal Electrolyte and Acid-Base, 175
Jody Nugent-Deal, RVT, VTS (Anesthesia/Analgesia &
Clinical Practice-Exotic Companion Animal)
and Stephen Cital, RVT, RLAT, SRA

Index, 207

List of Contributors

Brandee Bean
Adobe Animal Hospital
Los Altos
California, USA

Angela Chapman
Head Nurse Emergency and Critical Care
University of Melbourne Veterinary
Hospital Victoria, Australia

Stephen Cital
Director of Anaesthetic Nursing and
Training
United Veterinary Specialty and
Emergency
Interventionalist, Surpass Inc.
Relief Veterinary Technician, Oakland Zoo
Oakland
California, USA

Dave Cowan
Veterinary Technician
Veterinary Emergency Centre of Manchester
Manchester, UK

Meri Hall
Veterinary Specialty Hospital of Palm
Beach Gardens
Palm Beach Gardens
Florida, USA

Katherine Howie
Principal Nurse Manager
Vets Now-Emergency
UK

David Liss
Program Director-Veterinary Technology
Platt College
Los Angeles

Jody Nugent-Deal
Anaesthesia Department Supervisor
University of California Davis and
William R. Pritchard Veterinary Medical
Teaching Hospital
Instructor for VSPN.org,
VetMedTeam.com

Louise O'Dwyer
Clinical Support Manager
Vets Now Ltd
UK

Paula Plummer
Feline Internal Medicine Service
Texas A&M University Teaching Hospital
Texas, USA

Angela Randels-Thorp
Team Director
1st Pet Veterinary Centers
Arizona

Jo Woodison
Jo-Pet Emergency and Specialty Center
of Marin
San Rafael
California, USA

Eric Zamora-Moran
Small Animal Surgery Technologist
Supervisor
Purdue University Veterinary Teaching
Hospital
Indiana, USA

Foreword

It is gratifying for me to see Blackwell-Wiley's publication of this *Acid-Base and Electrolyte Handbook for Veterinary Technicians* by Angela Randels-Thorp and David Liss. This work clearly is more than a "handbook" in that the authors have taken care to explain the physiology and pathophysiology underlying disturbances in acid-base and electrolyte homeostasis. Their love of the subject shows in their treatment of it. As I previously said in the preface to my own textbook, *Fluid, Electrolyte, and Acid Base Disorders in Small Animal Practice*, a sound foundation in physiology and pathophysiology enables the clinician to best understand the abnormalities he or she encounters: "Thoughtful evaluation of laboratory results provides valuable insight into the fluid, electrolyte and acid base status of the animal and can only improve the veterinary care provided." The same can be said for veterinary technicians. If they understand the basis for the abnormal laboratory findings, they will be better able to take an informed approach to care for their veterinary patients. This type of in-depth understanding allows veterinarians and veterinary technicians to make the best decisions when treating their patients. A favorite example of mine is understanding why chloride is the critical electrolyte needed to restore acid base balance in a dog or cat with metabolic alkalosis caused by protracted vomiting of stomach contents (HINT: it involves the vital need of the kidneys to reabsorb sodium in the volume-depleted patient). Understanding the pathophysiology allows the clinician to make the logical choice of 0.9% NaCl as the crystalloid fluid of choice in this situation.

Randels-Thorp and Liss have taken an in-depth approach in their book, and indicate that they hope they are "providing an easy to understand approach to this detailed material, while not neglecting to incorporate the advanced nature of the topic." They have delivered on this promise in their book, which takes considerable care to explain the physiology behind the laboratory abnormalities. Their approach will be useful not only to veterinary technicians pursuing specialty certification but also to veterinary students and veterinarians too. Their book provides valuable information about disorders of sodium, chloride, potassium, calcium, magnesium, and phosphorus as well as acid base disorders. The authors have not shied away from complexity, and have included a chapter on mixed acid base disturbances as well as a chapter on the non-traditional approach to acid base balance, along with case examples to illustrate the value of the non-traditional approach in complicated cases. The final chapter (Companion Exotic Animal Electrolytes and Acid-Base) provides in one place hard-to-find valuable information not only about exotic mammalian species but also about birds, reptiles, and fish. I hope the community of veterinary technicians welcomes the challenge the authors have given them and uses this book as a foundation for advanced studies and specialty certification.

Stephen P. DiBartola,

DVM, ACVIM (internal medicine)

Emeritus Professor

Department of Veterinary Clinical Sciences

College of Veterinary Medicine

Ohio State University

Columbus, OH 43210

About the Companion Website

This book is accompanied by a companion website:

www.wiley.com/go/liss/electrolytes

The website includes:

- Interactive MCQs
- Case studies
- Figures

CHAPTER 1

Introduction to Acid-Base and Electrolytes

Angela Randels-Thorp, CVT, VTS (ECC, SAIM) and David Liss, RVT, VTS (ECC, SAIM)

Understanding of acid-base and electrolyte chemistry and physiology is both an important and valuable knowledge base for all veterinary technicians, and especially those in emergency and critical care or specialty practice. These very topics, however, are frequently thought of as boring at best or utterly confusing at worst. In actuality neither is true. These topics are often approached in a piecemeal or qualitative way, which lends itself to confusion. It is the goal of this text to provide a useful, easy-to-learn, and practical approach to the concepts regarding acid-base and electrolytes.

Introduction to acid-base

Assessment of acid-base status provides insight into three physiologic processes: alveolar ventilation, acid-base status, and oxygenation. Evaluating acid-base status has become an integral part of the emergent/critical care patient workup and should be performed as a baseline on all emergent patients. Deviation from normal acid-base balances is indicative of clinical disease processes and can aid the clinician in identifying underlying causes of illness in the patient. Venous samples can provide most of the information needed regarding acid-base status and even alveolar ventilation. Arterial samples are required, however, in order to provide oxygenation status (Sorrell-Raschi 2009). It is ever more important for the emergency and critical care (ECC) technician to be familiar in his/her understanding of acid-base values and what they mean.

Acid-Base and Electrolyte Handbook for Veterinary Technicians, First Edition.
Edited by Angela Randels-Thorp and David Liss.
© 2017 John Wiley & Sons, Inc. Published 2017 by John Wiley & Sons, Inc.
Companion website: www.wiley.com/go/liss/electrolytes

What is acidity?

In the simplest of terms, the acidity or alkalinity of a solution is based on how many hydrogen (H^+) ions, or molecules of carbon dioxide (CO_2), are present. Hydrogen ions are produced daily as a normal part of metabolism of protein and phospholipids, and are considered a fixed, non-volatile acid. Carbon dioxide is a byproduct of the metabolism of fat and carbohydrates in the body, and is considered a volatile acid (volatile = readily vaporized). Gaseous CO_2 is soluble in water. CO_2 is considered an acid because it readily combines with H_2O in the presence of carbonic anhydrase (enzyme/catalyst) to form carbonic acid (H_2CO_3). Without the catalyst, this change occurs very slowly. CO_2 is continually removed by ventilation and thereby kept at a stable partial pressure (pCO_2) in the body. The change in dissolved CO_2 in body fluids is proportional to pCO_2 in the gas phase. Elimination of these acids is dependent on the function of the lung, kidney, and liver.

Bronsted and Lowry state an acid is a proton donor (H^+) and a base is a proton acceptor (A^-) (DiBartola 2006: 229). The H^+ concentration ($[H^+]$) of body fluids must be kept at a constant level to prevent detrimental changes in enzyme function and cellular structure. Levels compatible with life are between 16 and 160 nEq/L. Excessive hydrogen ions in the blood result in acidemia. Decreased hydrogen ions in the blood result in alkalemia (Kovacic 2009). Hydrogen ions are not typically measured or tested in clinical practice. Therefore, Sorenson developed pH notation in order to provide simpler notation of the wide range of $[H^+]$ (DiBartola 2006: 229). There is an inverse relationship between pH and $[H^+]$ (Ex: $\uparrow[H^+] \rightarrow \downarrow pH$). Normal pH ranges between 7.35 and 7.45, approximately. The processes which lead to changes in production, retention, or excretion of acids or bases, which may or may not result in a change in pH, are called acidosis or alkalosis.

Buffering systems

The body contains several mechanisms in order to maintain the desired "normal" pH level, which is called buffering. A buffer is a compound that can accept or donate protons (H^+) and minimize a change in pH. Buffers consist of a weak acid and its conjugate salt (Sorrell-Raschi 2009). If a strong acid is added to a buffer, the protons from the acid dissociate to the salt of the buffer and the change of pH is therefore minimized. With these buffers the body is continually converting CO_2, H_2O, H^+, and HCO_3^- to maintain pH within normal ranges. The following equation represents this constant interaction:

$$CO_2 + H_2O \leftrightarrow H^+ + HCO_3^-$$

There are several compounds that serve as buffers in the body. The primary buffer of extracellular fluid (ECF) is bicarbonate (HCO_3^-). Non-bicarbonate buffers consist of proteins and inorganic and organic phosphates, which are primarily intracellular fluid (ICF) buffers. Bone is a prominent source of buffer (calcium carbonate and calcium phosphate). Up to 40% of buffering can be done from resources found in bone. Upon treatment/administration of sodium bicarbonate ($NaHCO_3^-$), carbonate that has been released to buffer can then be deposited back into the bone. In the blood, proteins, including hemoglobin and plasma, serve as buffers. Hemoglobin constitutes 80% of the buffering capacity of blood, whereas plasma proteins only account for 20% of buffering in the blood.

The body's buffering system is considered an open buffering system, with both bicarbonate and carbonic acid systems. In a closed system the exchanges would have to occur in a reciprocal manner. Since the body eliminates the majority of CO_2 through ventilation, keeping pCO_2 constant, a reciprocal reaction does not have to occur, which allows the body's buffering systems to be considered open. Both hydrogen ion excretion and bicarbonate regeneration are regulated by the kidneys.

Physiologic response system

The balance of acid-base in the body is regulated by metabolic, respiratory, and renal pathways. In terms of acid-base discussion, generally either a metabolic or a respiratory derangement occurs with the renal or respiratory system compensating for either/both.

When an excess of H^+ ions occurs, this causes a decrease in pH. Within minutes of this imbalance, the hydrogen ions begin to titrate with bicarbonate ions in ECF and then titrate with ICF buffers in order to minimize changes in pH. Next, alveolar ventilation is stimulated in order to decrease CO_2 until levels are below normal, thereby raising the pH back up to near normal. Within hours (2–3 days peak effect), the renal system begins to regenerate HCO_3^-. As HCO_3^- is increased, the body's pH is increased. Alveolar ventilation no longer needs to be increased, so returns to normal rates, restoring pCO_2 levels to normal.

CO_2 concentrations are a balance of mitochondrial production and alveolar removal by ventilation. An excess of CO_2 (in excess of ventilatory regulation) cannot be buffered directly by HCO_3^-. CO_2 is converted to carbonic acid by the mechanisms described above, which then allows H^+ from carbonic acid to titrate with intracellular buffers (proteins/phosphates). The renal system also adapts by increasing HCO_3^- reabsorption (2–5 days peak effect).

There is a variety of terms that can be used to describe acid-base imbalances, including: acidosis, alkalosis, acidemia, and alkalemia. While it may seem overly technical, knowing the differences between the terminologies can be important. The terms acidosis/alkalosis refer to the pathophysiologic processes that cause the net accumulation of acid or alkali in the body. The terms acidemia/alkalemia refer to the actual change in pH of ECF. In cases of acidemia, the pH is lower than normal, or <7.35 ($\uparrow[H^+]$). With alkalemia, the pH is higher than normal, or >7.45 ($\downarrow[H^+]$). For example: a patient with chronic respiratory acidosis may have normal pH due to renal compensation. The patient has acidosis, but not acidemia. Mixed acid-base disorders may also have an overall normal pH, due to one counter-balancing the other (Murtaugh 2002). These concepts will be covered in more detail in subsequent chapters.

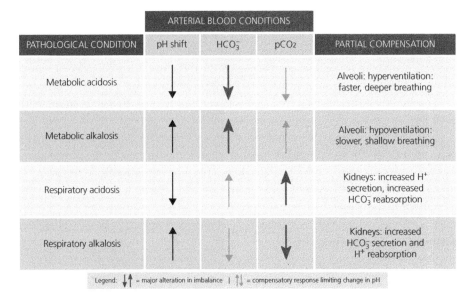

Figure 1.1 Arterial blood gases chart.

Primary acid-base disturbances

There are four primary acid-base disturbances that may occur in the body: metabolic acidosis, metabolic alkalosis, respiratory acidosis, and respiratory alkalosis. When evaluating a patient's acid-base status, the following parameters are primarily needed: pH, HCO_3^- (or TCO_2), and pCO_2 (Figure 1.1). If blood gases, or oxygenation, are being evaluated on an arterial blood sample, then PaO_2 values are also provided. Simple acid-base analysis may be done on either venous or arterial blood samples. Arterial samples are mandatory if one is attempting to assess the oxygenation status of a patient.

These imbalances will be discussed in greater detail throughout the chapters of this text, as well as practical approaches and applications for day-to-day practice.

Introduction to electrolytes

Just as fluid imbalances can affect the patient's electrolyte balance, electrolyte imbalances can, in turn, result in fluid imbalances, as well as a host of other problems. Imbalances involving sodium, potassium, chloride, calcium, phosphorus, and magnesium can all result in potentially life-threatening problems for animals. It is imperative for technicians to understand the role of electrolytes in the body and recognize the signs of imbalances in these electrolytes in order to aid in the quick recognition, diagnosis, and treatment of these problems. In this section we will introduce electrolyte physiology and regulation in the body, and specific and greater detail on each is covered in its respective chapter.

General electrolyte physiology (Table 1.1)

Electrolytes are substances that ionize when dissolved in ionizing solvents, such as water. An example would include salt, or sodium chloride (NaCl), which when dissolved in water ionizes to form Na^+ and Cl^- ions. A positively charged ion is called a cation (example Na^+) and a negatively charged ion is called an anion (example Cl^-). Electrolytes, in their ionic form, are extremely important in the body as they promote cardiac and neurologic impulse transmissions, regulate water balance, assist in skeletal muscle contraction, regulate acid-base balance, maintain oncotic balance (albumin), and provide concentration gradients for glomerular filtration in the kidney, among many other functions (Table 1.2).

Typically the body's electrolytes are distributed intra- and extracellularly, and it is important to understand in which compartment they mostly reside. Sodium, the body's primary and most abundant cation, resides extracellularly. In addition, sodium's counterpart, chloride, and bicarbonate reside mainly

Table 1.1 Common electrolytes and their charges

Name	Chemical symbol	Charge	Anion/Cation	Role in the body
Sodium	Na^+	1^+	Cation	Nervous/cardiac impulse transmission Water balance
Chloride	Cl^-	1^-	Anion	Water balance Acid-base balance
Potassium	K^+	1^+	Cation	Nervous/cardiac impulse transmission
Magnesium	Mg^{2+}	2^+	Cation	Co-factor in enzymatic processes
Phosphorus/Phosphate	PO_4^{3-}	3^-	Anion	Acid-base buffer Biochemical reactions
Bicarbonate	HCO_3^-	1^-	Anion	Acid-base buffer
Calcium	Ca^{2+}	2^+	Cation	Skeletal/cardiac muscle contraction
Lactate	CH_3CHCO_2H	1^-	Anion	Byproduct of anaerobic metabolism

Table 1.2 Average intracellular/extracellular electrolyte concentrations

Electrolyte	Average serum concentration (mEq/L)	Average intracellular concentration (mEq/L)
Sodium	142	12
Potassium	4.3	140
Chloride	104	4
Bicarbonate	24	12
Magnesium	1.1	34
Phosphate	2.0	40
Calcium	2.5	4

extracellularly. The abundant intracellular electrolytes include: potassium, calcium, magnesium, and phosphorus/phosphate.

Units of measure

Electrolytes are typically measured in mEq/L, or milliequivalent weight per liter, but can also be expressed as mg/dL or milligrams per deciliter. The milliequivalent weight (or mEq/L) represents the atomic, molecular, or formula weight of a substance divided by its valence. The valence number of a substance refers to the net number of charges it accumulates when it ionizes. For example, calcium, as Ca^{2+}, would have a valence of 2; chloride, as Cl^-, would have a valence of 1. Using sodium as an example, since it has a 1^+ charge its valence number is 1. That means each millimole of sodium provides 1 mEq of sodium, because we are dividing the ionic weight by 1. Atomic, molecular, and formula weights and other units of measure are summarized in Table 1.3. In the case of magnesium, because its valence number is 2, each millimole would contribute in reality 0.5 mEq because we would divide by a valence of 2. This simply provides a reasonable unit of measure when dealing with substances that exist in very large quantities in the body. As some electrolytes are typically measured or reported in concentrations

Table 1.3 Units of measurement of electrolytes

Unit of measure	Definition
Atomic mass Example: $^{12}C = 12.000$	Unitless measure of weight which is an average of all the isotopic weights of a substance. It is typically reported in the periodic table of the elements. For example, C is typically reported as ^{12}C and weighs 12.000
Molecular mass Example: $H_{2O} = 18$	The weight of a molecule (combination of atoms) represented by the addition of their combined atomic weights. For example: H_2O has a molecular mass of 18 because O has an atomic mass of 16 and H has an atomic mass of 1 (which is doubled by the presence of two H molecules)
Formula weight Example: $CaCl_2 = 111$	This is similar to molecular mass but typically is discussed in the case of ions. Since ions dissociate in a solvent, this term is used. Example: calcium chloride is $CaCl_2$ and has a formula weight of 111. This comes from calcium's weight of $40 + 2 \times$ chloride's weight of 35.5
Mole	A unit of measure for a large number of particles. 6.02×10^{23} particles of a substance = 1 mole of that substance
Molar mass	This term refers to the weight in grams of 1 mole of a substance. For example, 1 mole of sodium (which is 6.02×10^{23} sodium ions) weighs 23 grams
Millimole/milligram	This represents one-thousandth (10^{-3}) of a mole or a gram
Valence Example: Ca^{2+} = valence of 2	A number representing the number of charges an ion has. Example: Ca^{2+} has a valence of 2; Cl^- has a valence of 1
Milliequivalent (mEq)	This is a measure of an ion's millimolecular weight divided by its valence

(such as mg/dL) these units can be converted back and forth. Phosphorus has an approximately normal plasma concentration of 4 mg/dL. Its average valence, because it exists in several forms, is 1.8. The molecular weight of phosphorus is 31. The equation to convert mg/dL to mEq/L is:

$$\frac{mEq}{L} = \frac{\dfrac{mg}{dL} \times 10}{molecular\ weight} \times valence$$

So our equation becomes:

$$\frac{mEq}{L} = \frac{4 \times 10}{31} \times 1.8 = 2.3\,mEq/L$$

Although not terribly important to commit to memory, a basic understanding of the units used to report electrolytes is essential in forming a foundation for interpreting them clinically.

Osmolality and osmolarity

A fundamental concept in electrolyte physiology is understanding how electro-lytes affect fluid movement across membranes (tissue, cellular, etc.). This is described in the concept of osmolality. Osmolality describes the number of osmoles per kilogram of solvent, and osmolarity represents the number of osmoles per liter of solvent. An osmole is a measure of the solutes in a solution that exert an osmotic effect and typically is represented as 1 Osm is equal to 1 gram of molecular weight, which also indicates 6.02×10^{23} particles from the definition of a mol. This would be the case of a molecule that does not dissociate in the solution. In the case of NaCl, which dissociates into Na^+ and Cl^-, a millimole of NaCl would contribute 2 mOsm (milliosmole) (1 mOsm of Na^+ and 1 mOsm of Cl^-). In biologic fluids osmolarity and osmolality are used interchangeably and for the sake of uniformity osmolality will be used going forward in this chapter.

The total osmolarity of a solution represents the number of osmoles present in a solution. This can be measured in serum in a clinical patient and is typically between 300 and 310 mOsm/kg in the dog and cat. Hyper- and hypo-osmolar conditions can arise and are beyond the scope of this chapter but will be discussed in future chapters in this textbook.

Since osmoles exert an osmotic effect, they can affect fluid balance and movement in a solution with a membrane. Osmosis is defined as a spontaneous movement of a solvent (fluid) across a semi-permeable membrane from a region of lower solute concentration (solid) to a region of higher solute con-centration. This movement will cause an equilibrium in the concentrations of solutes on either side. For example, imagine a beaker with a thin membrane dividing it into two halves. One each side there is a solvent (liquid) of equal volume, and one adds sodium chloride (salt) to the right side. Now on the right

Ineffective osmole

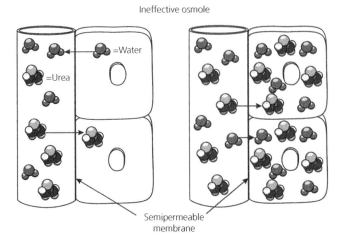

Effective osmole

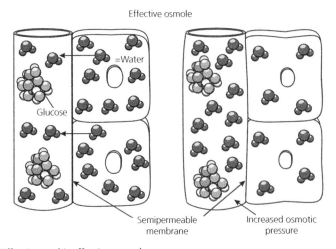

Figure 1.2 Effective and ineffective osmoles.

side there is much solute compared to the left side and this means it is highly concentrated on the right and dilute (low concentration) on the left. Thus, the water will move from the diluted left side (with more solvent than solute) to the more concentrated right side (with more solute than solvent) creating an equilibrium of solute:solvent on each side. This is depicted in the upper portion of Figure 1.2.

This concept is extremely important in physiology, as the body has several of these membranes. Of note are the cellular membrane and the capillary membrane. For a thorough discussion of the anatomy of these, the reader is directed to a physiology textbook, but water and fluid must remain outside of a cell, inside of a cell, outside of a capillary (in tissue) and inside a capillary (blood volume) in appropriate proportions or disease ensues.

Also, not all osmoles are created equal. Some, although called osmoles, can traverse a physiologic membrane and thus do not exert an osmotic effect. These are called ineffective osmoles and lie in contrast to effective osmoles that will pull the solvent across the membrane. An example of an ineffective osmoles is urea: where urea could exert an osmotic effect in the laboratory, in the body urea can pass through the pores of a semi-permeable cellular membrane thereby creating an equilibrium of solute, causing no net movement of solvent across the membrane. This is demonstrated in the lower portion of Figure 1.2. Effective osmoles have a special name for their measure in bodily fluids. This is referred to as the tonicity. The tonicity of a solution is the measure of the effective osmolarity. So in a solution with tonicity fluid will move across the semi-permeable membrane when an effective osmole is added. One such example is sodium. Sodium is an effective osmole in the body, and solutions where there is more sodium relative to the concentration of solvent are referred to as hypertonic, and solutions where the solute (sodium) concentration is less than the solvent are called hypotonic. When solvent:solute concentrations are equal that is called an isotonic solution.

Fluid movement across bodily compartments/membranes

In order to fully understand disorders of sodium and chloride, the veterinary technician needs to comprehend the idea of fluid movement across membranes that reside in the body. Fluid is maintained in several different compartments, including the ICF compartment and the ECF compartment. The ECF compartment is then divided into interstitial fluid (ISF) and intravascular fluid (IVF) compartments. The cell membrane divides the ICF and the ECF compartments and the capillary membrane divides the IVF from the ISF compartments. Osmotically active particles will largely determine the fluid balance across the cell membrane which maintains the balance between the ICF and ECF compartments. In this case, these effective osmoles are not easily or at all permeable to the cell membrane and thus exert the concentration effect drawing fluid either in or out of the cell across the membrane. Sodium, potassium, chloride, bicarbonate, glucose, and to some extent urea can all affect osmolality and fluid balance. Gain or loss of these osmoles from the extracellular or intracellular space, or gain or loss of fluid on either side, will create a ripple effect, causing net movement of fluid in or out of the cell across the cell membrane. Further descriptions of these effects are found later in this textbook.

Movement of fluid across the capillary membrane is quite different. Although not fully understood, the idea of Starling's forces remains the major theory to describe net fluid movement from the interstitial space into or out of the capillary or into and out of the tissue space. Starling's equation is:

$$\text{Net filtration} = K_f \left[\left(P_{cap} - P_{if} \right) - \left(\pi_{cap} - \pi_{if} \right) \right]$$

While seemingly daunting at first, this equation simply describes how fluid moves across the capillary membrane. The net filtration, if positive, means fluid extravasates out of the capillary and if negative means fluid moves into the capillary.

K_f = Filtration coefficient, describes the permeability of the capillary wall

P_{cap} = The hydrostatic pressure inside the capillary (fluid pressure), will tend to drive fluid out of the capillary if elevated

P_{if} = The hydrostatic pressure of the tissues, will tend to drive fluid into the capillary if elevated

π_{cap} = The oncotic pressure in the capillary. This is the pressure generated by plasma proteins (negatively charged) attracting water toward them and thus tending to draw water into the capillary and keeping it there.

π_{if} = Represents the oncotic pressure in the tissues. This tends to exert a pressure maintaining water inside the tissue (interstitial) space.

Disturbances in Starling's law demonstrate why fluid would move out of the capillary space, causing edema, or potentially into the capillary space, causing hypervolemia. If the capillary hydrostatic pressure increases, as caused by congestive heart failure in pulmonary capillaries, water will tend to move out of the capillary and into the interstitial space, thus causing pulmonary edema. If plasma protein concentration drops, such as in hypoproteinemia or hypoalbuminemia, the capillary oncotic pressure drops as well. As this pressure tends to maintain water within the capillary space, when it is not present water will tend to leak out of the capillary and into the tissue bed, also causing edema.

The anion gap

The anion gap is a concept that will be discussed in later chapters in reference to acid-base. As electrolytes have charges and affect fluid balance, disturbances in them can be responsible for causing acid-base conditions. The anion gap can help identify if certain electrolytes are responsible for the acid-base condition, or illuminate other causes. The body exists in a state of electroneutrality, meaning all electrolyte charges sum to zero. All cation charges (positive) when added to all anion charges (negative) are equal and thus maintain a 0 net charge in the body. However, routine analyzers don't measure all known anions and cations. So trying to identify total concentrations of all electrolytes becomes challenging. For example, only sodium and potassium, and chloride and bicarbonate, are routinely measured. Even if phosphorus, magnesium, and lactate are measured, there are still ions that are unaccounted for. Due to limits of technology, analyzers tend to analyze more cations than anions, meaning more anions are not measured in clinical assays. This leads to an overabundance of anion charges/

measures that are not accounted for routinely. If unmeasured anions (UAs) and unmeasured cations (UCs) are represented in a total neutrality equation, one can develop an equation accounting for these unmeasured, yet biologically active, ions.

1 Total cations should equal total anions: $Na^+ + K^+ + UC = Cl^- + HCO_3^- + UA$

2 Rearranging: Measured cations – measured anions = UA – UC = anion gap

3 Final: $(Na^+ + K^+) - (Cl^- + HCO_3^-) = UA - UC$

   The result of the third equation will yield a number representing how many more UAs there are than UCs. For example, if lactate (typically a UA) is high, it will make the UA value in the third equation much higher, yielding an elevated anion gap. More on this in later chapters.

Fluid maintenance and loss basics

Although mainly about electrolytes and acid-base, this textbook will cover some measure of discussion on fluids, fluid balance, and gain or loss in the presence of disease. As electrolytes affect fluid balance across compartments, as discussed above, alterations in gain or loss of fluid will also exert osmotic and fluid-moving effects.

   Typically, the body exists in a state of equilibrium of fluid movement, called homeostasis. Fluid is lost and gained in equal proportions to maintain hydration and blood volume. All gains and losses end up totaling to zero, meaning no net gain or loss. A gain of fluid is called a positive fluid balance and a loss of fluid is called a negative fluid balance. These can occur in disease states.

   Fluid or water loss is described as sensible or insensible. Sensible losses are those that can be measured or quantified easily, and insensible losses are those that must be estimated. Water lost in urine, feces, or saliva is typically called sensible loss and can be measured. Insensible losses include sweating and evaporative losses from the skin and respiratory tract.

   Water lost through the kidney (sensible urinary water loss) can take two forms: water with solute (called obligatory water loss), which helps maintain solute balance in the kidney and body, and water without solute (simply H_2O, also called free water loss) which is generated through the action of vasopressin/antidiuretic hormone (ADH) on the kidney. Remember the examples of sodium and water in a beaker with a membrane? The loss of water through the kidney can effectively change sodium or water concentrations in the body. If water and sodium are lost in equal proportions through the kidney (obligatory water loss), all concentrations remain the same. But if free water (simply H_2O) is lost, a concentration gradient is established because the water on one side of the membrane (in this case outside of the cell) is depleted of water but still has sodium. This becomes a hypertonic solution. The same situation could occur if water was lost in great amounts through respiratory or evaporative means. This will cause disease in the body and will be discussed in more detail in later chapters.

Conclusion

Understanding these general concepts of acid-base balance and electrolyte/fluid physiology in the body are essential to move on to later chapters in this text. The veterinary technician cannot understand hypertonic fluid loss in the presence of hypernatremia, or hyperosmolar states or triple acid-base disorders without first mastering the basic physiologic concepts discussed here. Once these concepts are fully understood, alterations in electrolyte or acid-base balance will make sense and allow the veterinary technician to fully comprehend the complex physiologic alterations occurring during the disease conditions. Although confusing and sometimes frustrating, having a strong foundation in electrolyte and acid-base conditions is essential for the veterinary technician working with sick and injured patients. Electrolyte and acid-base abnormalities affect all species, ages, breeds, and disease conditions and can cause life-threatening alterations in heart rate, cardiac conduction, blood pressure, and nervous transmission. The veterinary technician must be ready to quickly identify abnormalities, alert the attending veterinarian, and apply rapid treatment to stabilize the critically ill veterinary patient.

References

DiBartola, S. (2006). Introduction to acid-base disorders. In: S. DiBartola (ed.), *Fluid, Electrolytes, and Acid-Base Disorders in Small Animal Practice*, 3rd ed. St Louis, MO: Saunders Elsevier.

Kovacic, J. (2009). Acid-base disturbances. In: D. C. Silverstein & K. Hopper (eds), *Small Animal Critical Care Medicine*. St Louis, MO: Saunders Elsevier: 249–54.

Murtaugh, R. (2002). *Quick Look Series in Veterinary Medicine-Critical Care*. Jackson, WY: Teton New Media, Chapter 14.

Sorrell-Raschi, L. (2009). Blood gas and oximetry monitoring. In: D. C. Silverstein & K. Hopper (eds), *Small Animal Critical Care Medicine*. St Louis, MO: Saunders Elsevier: 878–82.

CHAPTER 2
Disorders of Sodium

Angela Chapman, BSc (Hons), RVN, Dip HE CVN, Dip AVN, VTS (ECC)

Sodium is an extremely important electrolyte in the body and is routinely measured in both baseline testing and ongoing monitoring of sick patients. It is easily measured using a wide range of point of care or laboratory analyzers and is expressed as milliequivalents or millimoles per liter of plasma (mEq/L or mmol/L respectively). Normal extracellular fluid (ECF) levels of sodium are approximately 140 mEq/L, whereas sodium levels in the intracellular fluid (ICF) are only about 10 mEq/L. As the body's major extracellular cation (positively charged ion), sodium has several key functions, including:
- maintaining water homeostasis, including volume and distribution of water within the body;
- contributing to impulse transmission in nerve and muscle fibers;
- maintaining cellular electroneutrality.

Disorders of sodium can be relatively common in critically ill animals and severe derangements can lead to the development of neurologic issues. Treatment is not always easy, or straightforward, and if not initiated carefully can lead to development or worsening of existing neurologic signs, and in some cases death. Therefore, a thorough knowledge of the complex factors influencing the physiologic causes of sodium derangements and how these impact treatment are imperative to the successful management of these patients.

Physiology

Sodium balance is closely linked to water homeostasis. Though sodium and water are regulated by different mechanisms, the result has an impact on both, and therefore it is important to understand both processes in order to appreciate the role and balance of sodium in the body.

Acid-Base and Electrolyte Handbook for Veterinary Technicians, First Edition.
Edited by Angela Randels-Thorp and David Liss.
© 2017 John Wiley & Sons, Inc. Published 2017 by John Wiley & Sons, Inc.
Companion website: www.wiley.com/go/liss/electrolytes

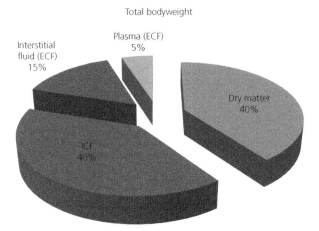

Figure 2.1 Distribution of water by total bodyweight.

Approximately 60% of normal adult bodyweight is water. Two-thirds (40% of bodyweight) of this water is found in the cells of the body and is referred to as the ICF compartment. The remaining third (20% of bodyweight) is found in the ECF compartment and distributed between the interstitial fluid (75% of ECF, 15% of bodyweight) that bathes the cells, and plasma (25% of ECF, 5% of bodyweight) (Wellman, DiBartola, & Kohn 2012; Figure 2.1). Water moves relatively easily between these compartments, and its distribution is established and maintained by the osmolality of plasma, which, in large part, is due to sodium concentration.

Osmoles are particles dissolved in a solution that contribute to the pull of water across a cell membrane, a process known as osmosis. Osmolality is a measure of the *number* of osmoles per kilogram of solvent. This measurement does not take into account the weight, charge, or size of the osmoles, merely the quantity. Water will flow along a concentration gradient from an area of low osmolality (few particles) to an area of high osmolality (many particles) until the concentration of osmoles is equal. This is also known as osmotic pressure. Osmoles can be categorized as *effective* or *ineffective* depending on their size and ability to freely cross a semi-permeable membrane. Effective osmoles are too large to easily cross a semi-permeable membrane and therefore influence the movement of water by drawing it across the cell membrane to establish equilibrium.

Sodium is the primary effective osmole of the ECF (Wellman, DiBartola, & Kohn 2012). It is pumped out of the ICF in exchange for potassium, which is the primary effective osmole of the ICF. This occurs by a process known as active transport via the sodium-potassium adenosine triphosphatase pump (Na^+/K^+-ATPase). This pump is a protein found in the membrane of all cells and utilizes energy in the form of ATP to actively move sodium molecules out of cells and potassium molecules into cells against their concentration gradients. As a consequence, the sodium levels outside of the cell are substantially higher than inside,

Table 2.1 Distribution of sodium and potassium in the intra-extracellular fluid (Source: Adapted from Guyton & Hall 2011)

	ICF	ECF
Sodium (mEq/L)	14	142
Potassium (mEq/L)	140	4

and the opposite is seen with potassium (Table 2.1). This process is essential to maintain the resting membrane potential (or electroneutrality) of the cell, and is important for a number of physiologic functions, including generation of action potentials in the transmission of nerve impulses and active transport of a number of substances across cell membranes (Guyton & Hall 2011).

Measured sodium reflects the volume of sodium in the plasma, which is representative of the sodium levels across the ECF. The remaining sodium in the body is found in small volumes in the ICF, or in bone as insoluble salts. Sodium contained in bones cannot be exchanged or utilized by fluid compartments in the body and therefore does not contribute to sodium imbalances that may occur. (Wellman, DiBartola, & Kohn 2012).

Because water and sodium are so closely linked through the body's requirement to maintain osmotic equilibrium, plasma or serum sodium measurements must be considered in relation to the amount of water in the ECF. A low plasma sodium concentration could reflect a true decrease in ECF sodium volume, or a normal sodium volume diluted in an abnormally high volume of plasma water creating a relative decrease.

Sodium and water balance

The body has a number of complex feedback mechanisms in place in order to maintain tight control over sodium and water levels in the body. Sodium balance occurs primarily in the kidney and it is important to understand how and where this occurs in order to appreciate the effect of other influencing factors, such as drugs and disease states.

Sodium retention

Under normal circumstances, the kidneys excrete only the volume of sodium that is ingested each day in order to maintain a tightly controlled balance. Sodium is filtered by the glomeruli of the kidneys and the vast majority of it is reabsorbed throughout the renal tubules in order to maintain balanced body sodium levels. This process is assisted by various pumps in the cells lining the tubular membrane, or wall of the renal tubule. On the basolateral membrane (surface of the tubular wall that is directed outward toward the interstitium), cell walls contain basolateral sodium-potassium pumps (Figure 2.2). These pump sodium out of the tubular membrane and into the interstitial fluid in order to

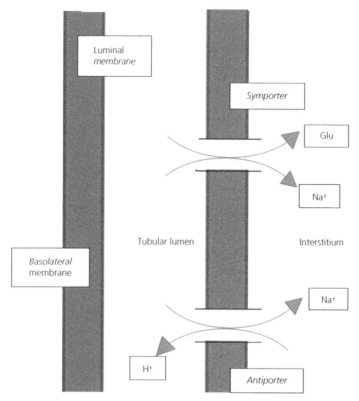

Figure 2.2 Transport of sodium across the luminal membrane of the renal tubule through the use of membrane co-transporter proteins.

create a concentration gradient to facilitate the reabsorption of sodium. The luminal (or apical) membrane (surface of the tubular wall that is directed inward toward the inner lumen of the renal tubule) contains a variety of membrane co-transporter proteins that facilitate the transport of two coupled molecules across a membrane. These vary depending on the location in the renal tubule and the molecules to be transported.

Reabsorption across the luminal membrane occurs at four main sites:

- **Proximal convoluted tubule (PCT):** Approximately 67% of sodium is reabsorbed here (DiBartola 2012). This is achieved initially through symporters and latterly through antiporters. Symporters are a type of membrane co-transporter protein. One molecule, in this case sodium, moves *down* a concentration gradient and assists the transport of a coupled glucose molecule *up* a concentration gradient crossing the luminal (inner) membrane in the same direction (Figure 2.2). Later in the PCT, sodium utilizes antiporter membrane proteins, which exchange one molecule for another, moving them in opposite directions, with sodium being reabsorbed in exchange for hydrogen ions.
- **Thick ascending limb of the loop of Henle (LoH):** This is responsible for approximately 25% of filtered sodium (DiBartola 2012). Here the

sodium-hydrogen antiporter is utilized along with a different co-transporter that moves sodium, potassium, and chloride across the luminal membrane together.

- **Distal convoluted tubule (DCT):** A further 5% of sodium is reabsorbed here (DiBartola 2012) via a sodium-chloride co-transporter.
- **Collecting duct:** The remaining 3% of sodium is reabsorbed here (DiBartola 2012) through luminal sodium channels.

Sodium regulation

There are a number of different mechanisms in place to keep sodium under tight control. As sodium is so closely linked to water balance, this control is not only subject to direct detection of changes in sodium levels but also in response to an increase or decrease in circulating volume, which may be secondary to changes in sodium levels.

Responses to increased plasma sodium

Thirst response

One of the simplest physiologic responses to a true or relative increase in plasma sodium is the thirst response. This is triggered by osmoreceptors, which are sensory receptors, in the hypothalamus of the brain. These receptors detect tiny changes in the osmolality of plasma, as small as 1–2% (Robertson 1983). The osmoreceptors shrink in response to increases in plasma osmolality and swell as plasma osmolality decreases and the fluid becomes more dilute. When the osmoreceptors shrink, this triggers a physiologic urge to drink water, which will then increase water volume in the ECF and dilute the overall sodium plasma level.

Vasopressin (anti-diuretic hormone)

Vasopressin is a peptide hormone that is produced in the hypothalamus and released into the bloodstream from the posterior pituitary. Its release is stimulated by a reduction in circulating volume or an increase in plasma osmolality. This is detected in two ways:

- *Osmoreceptors* in the hypothalamus detect changes in osmolality and stimulate secretion of vasopressin at the same time as triggering the thirst response, as described above.
- *Baroreceptors* are sensory neurons found in the walls of blood vessels in the aortic arch and carotid sinus. They respond to stretching of the vessel wall, and thus detect changes in pressure within the vessels. Decrease in blood pressure stimulates the release of vasopressin.

The primary role of vasopressin is to increase blood pressure by increasing water reabsorption in the kidneys. It binds to V2 receptors in the principal cells of the collecting ducts and activates the insertion of aquaporin 2 channels into the luminal cell membranes of the collecting ducts. These channels facilitate the reabsorption of water and so their number is directly proportional to the volume of water reabsorbed. In the absence of vasopressin, these channels are removed by endocytosis, thereby reducing the volume of water reabsorbed (DiBartola 2012).

On a smaller scale, vasopressin can also contribute to vasoconstriction, which further aids to increase the blood pressure. In high concentrations it binds to V1 receptors in the vascular endothelial cells; however, this effect is generally not seen in the normal homeostatic response.

Responses to decreased plasma sodium
Renin–angiotensin–aldosterone system

A crucial system for maintaining sodium and water balance is the renin–angiotensin–aldosterone system (RAAS; Figure 2.3). This control originates in the juxtaglomerular apparatus (JGA) of the kidney, a structure found in each nephron comprising juxtaglomerular cells and the macula densa.

- The juxtaglomerular cells are specialized smooth muscle cells found in the afferent arterioles of the glomerulus. They are sensitive to changes in blood pressure, and respond to decreases in blood pressure, by releasing the enzyme renin into the circulation.

- Simultaneously, the glomerular filtration rate (GFR) slows in response to reduced blood pressure in the afferent (ingoing) arterioles. This reduction in filtration rate leads to an increase in sodium reabsorption along the PCT and the LoH.

- The macula densa cells make up the second part of the JGA and are a group of specialized cells that function as chemoreceptors. They are found at the junction of the ascending limb of the LoH and the DCT and detect changes in sodium concentration. When a reduction in sodium is detected (due to enhanced reabsorption in the PCT as a result of reduced GFR), these cells release nitric oxide and prostaglandins (Schricker, Hamann, & and Kurtz 1995), which cause vasodilation of the afferent arterioles in an effort to increase GFR and stimulate further release of renin by the juxtaglomerular cells.

- Baroreceptors in the carotid sinus also respond to a drop in blood pressure and stimulate the glossopharyngeal nerve (cranial nerve IX) sending a signal to the central nervous system (CNS; Stephenson 2007). The vasomotor center in the brain stimulates the sympathetic nervous system's (SNS) outflow from the renal medulla to the JGA, and norepinephrine is released which stimulates further release of renin from the juxtaglomerular cells.

- Renin is released into the circulation and hydrolyzes the plasma protein angiotensinogen, which is constantly produced by the liver. This converts angiotensinogen into a decapeptide angiotensin-1.

- Angiotensin-1 passes through the pulmonary circulation and is converted into an octapeptide angiotensin-2 by angiotensin-converting enzyme (ACE), which is produced by the endothelial cells in the pulmonary beds.

- Angiotensin-2 has a number of effects that bring about the restoration of euvolemia and normal sodium levels.

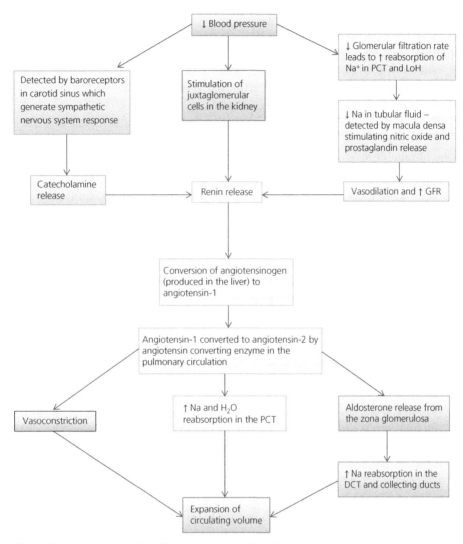

Figure 2.3 Renin-angiotensin-aldosterone system (RAAS).

1 Restoration of circulating volume through vasoconstriction, through increasing preload, thereby increasing stroke volume and cardiac output leading to an overall increase in systemic blood pressure.

2 Increases sodium reabsorption in the PCT through stimulation of the sodium-hydrogen antiporters.

3 Stimulates release of aldosterone from the zona glomerulosa in the adrenal cortex. Aldosterone upregulates the basolateral sodium-potassium pumps in the membrane of the DCT, and increases the number of sodium transporter channels in the luminal membrane. This creates a concentration gradient, thereby increasing sodium and water reabsorption in the DCT and collecting ducts.

Atrial natriuretic peptide (ANP)

ANP is a peptide hormone that is produced and stored in the atrial myocytes. It is released in response to an increase in circulating volume detected by baroreceptors in the cardiac atria and pulmonary vessels. As such, it works in the opposite scenario to vasopressin and aldosterone and acts to reduce water and sodium reabsorption when blood pressure is increased.

ANP increases GFR by dilating the afferent (ingoing) glomerular arterioles and dilating the efferent (outgoing) arterioles, thereby increasing the volume and filtration pressure within the glomerulus. It also relaxes the mesangial cells, which are the smooth muscle cells surrounding the blood vessels in the glomerulus. This increases the surface area available for filtration, thereby increasing sodium and water excretion. The increased blood flow also results in a reduction in the number of solutes in the interstitial fluid, which leads to decreased reabsorption of water and sodium in the PCT due to the reduced concentration gradient required for reabsorption.

It also reduces reabsorption of water and sodium in the DCT and collecting ducts through interaction with the co-transporters that are utilized in the luminal cells.

Finally, ANP directly inhibits renin and aldosterone secretion, thereby inhibiting the RAAS and its effects.

Clinical assessment of sodium derangements

When initially assessing a patient with a sodium derangement, a thorough evaluation of the patient's hydration status should also be completed (DiBartola 2012). This should comprise as a minimum:

- detailed history, including diet, any recent urination or drinking changes, any vomiting or diarrhea, and any other known medical conditions or current medications;
- thorough physical examination, including heart rate, respiratory rate and effort, pulse quality, skin turgor, capillary refill time, mucous membrane moistness, and mentation;
- diagnostic tests, including packed cell volume (PCV), total solids (TS), urine specific gravity (USG), glucose and blood pressure.

These will help to build a picture of the current overall hydration status of the patient, the potential underlying cause(s) of the sodium derangement, and the duration and extent of the condition. This information is essential to determine the classification of the derangement as well as the type and duration of treatment to be provided.

Hyponatremia

Hyponatremia describes sodium levels below 140 mEq/L (Nelson, Delaney, & Elliot 2009). Despite sodium being the main extracellular cation and being heavily involved in determination of osmolality, hyponatremia is not always associated with low plasma osmolality. Hyponatremia is divided into three categories; hypo-osmolar, normo-osmolar, and hyperosmolar.

In order to determine which category a patient falls into, the first step is to calculate the osmolality of the plasma. Plasma osmolality is determined by the presence of effective osmoles, as described previously in this chapter. Normal plasma osmolality is described as 300 mOsm/kg in the dog and 310 mOsm/kg in the cat (Wellman, DiBartola, & Kohn 2012). To calculate plasma osmolarity in the absence of a colloid osmometer, a simple equation can be used to estimate the value based on the major contributing osmoles:

$$\text{Plasma osmolality} = 2 \times \text{Na} + \left(\text{BUN}/2.8\right) + \left(\text{glucose}/18\right)$$

In the ECF these comprise sodium, chloride, glucose, and blood urea nitrogen (BUN). This formula calculates the combined total of these, with a factor of 2 for sodium to account for minor and immeasurable osmoles. The BUN and glucose are divided by separate factors to convert them from mg/dl to mmol/l (Burton & Theodore 2001). Once the osmolality has been determined, further aspects can be considered in order to establish the true etiology.

Normo-osmolar hyponatremia
Etiology
Normo-osmolar hyponatremia is also referred to as "pseudohyponatremia" or "factitious hyponatremia." It is seen as a result of a laboratory analyzer's error in older machines that utilize flame photometry to determine sodium levels. In the presence of extremely high levels of lipids or proteins, these analyzers overestimate the proportion of plasma present in the blood sample and consequently miscalculate the volume of sodium, giving a reading that is lower than it truly is. This error is not seen in more modern analyzers that utilize direct ion-selective electrodes to measure sodium (Nelson, Delaney, & Elliot 2009; DiBartola 2012).

Clinical signs
Clinical signs related to hyponatremia are not seen, as it is not a true hyponatremia. Visual evidence of hyperlipidemia in the blood sample may be seen, or excessively high serum protein levels may be found during further testing.

Treatment
Treatment is aimed at correcting the hyperlipidemia or hyperproteinemia, which will result in normalization of sodium measurements.

Nursing care/monitoring
Monitoring involves ascertaining a true plasma sodium value from a direct ion selective electrode analyzer to ensure that it is within the normal range. Additional nursing care will be based around treatment of the underlying cause.

Hyperosmolar hyponatremia
Etiology
Hyperosmolar hyponatremia is also known as "translocational hyponatremia" and is seen as a result of dilution of sodium due to the addition of an impermeant solute (solutes that cannot easily cross a semipermeable membrane) to the ECF, such as glucose (Bohn 2012). Glucose is an effective osmole; therefore high levels of glucose in the ECF draws more water from the ICF to maintain equilibrium between the two compartments. As a result, the plasma sodium is diluted, causing a secondary hyponatremia. This is most commonly seen in patients suffering from diabetes mellitus where an increase in plasma glucose is seen (DiBartola 2012). Hyperglycemic-hyperosmolar syndrome (HHS) is a complication of diabetes mellitus that can have a severe effect on plasma osmolality. This is characterized by severe hyperglycemia (>600 mg/dl) and hyperosmolality (>340 mOsm/kg) without the presence of ketones that would be seen in diabetic ketoacidosis (Koenig 2009). The effect that glucose has on sodium in these patients depends on the extent of glucose elevation. Studies in humans have shown that for every 100 mg/dl increase in glucose the plasma sodium decreases by 1.6 mEq/L up to a concentration of 440 mg/dl, after which it decreases at a much higher rate (Hillier, Abbott, & Barrett 1999). Therefore in order to calculate the corrected sodium level the following formula should be used:

$$Corrected\ Na^+ = Plasma\ Na^+ + 1.6*([Plasma\ glucose - normal\ glucose]/100)$$

*where the plasma glucose is >500 mg/dl a correction factor of 2.4 should be used instead of 1.6.

When corrected sodium levels are calculated in these patients they are often found to actually be normo-, or hypernatremic instead of hyponatremic. This should be taken into account during treatment. Hyperosmolar hyponatremia can also be seen with mannitol administration, which has the same osmotic effect as glucose.

Clinical signs
Clinical signs related to hyperosmolality include neurologic signs, such as circling, pacing, mentation changes, and seizures (Nelson, Delaney, & Elliot 2009; Guyton & Hall 2011). Typically plasma osmolarity must be >340 mmol/L for neurologic signs to appear. These signs develop due to the movement of water out of the ICF in response to the increased presence of effective osmoles in the ECF to establish equilibrium. As a result of this water movement, cells in the brain shrink and subsequent neurologic signs develop.

In cases that are not severe or acute enough to cause dehydration of brain cells, clinical signs will be related to the underlying condition.

Treatment

Primary treatment should be aimed at addressing the underlying cause. Hyper-osmolality and dehydration as a consequence of osmotic diuresis should be corrected. Fluid selection and rate of administration must be carefully evaluated in these patients. Osmolarity should be reduced at a rate of no more than 0.5 mEq/L/hr, or 10–12 mEq/L/24 hr. This is because the body responds to protect the brain from dehydration by making idiogenic osmoles to maintain cerebral water balance, similar to what happens in hypernatremic conditions. This is important to remember when starting treatment on these patients. When starting intravenous fluids (IVF), caution must be taken not to lower the osmolarity too quickly or risk the potential to cause cerebral edema. As osmolarity normalizes, sodium will automatically normalize. Laboratory testing every 2 hr is needed to recalculate osmolarity to ensure it is not changing too quickly. (Note: if glucose levels are above range of an analyzer, samples must be diluted to achieve an end point number in order to correctly calculate plasma osmolality initially, and throughout treatment.) Fluid selection should be based on the corrected sodium level and an isotonic fluid containing sodium levels closest to the patient's corrected sodium should be used.

Nursing care/monitoring

Nursing care should be aimed at monitoring the hydration and neurologic status of the patient as corrective treatments are initiated. Hydration and volume status should be monitored through regular assessment of respiratory rate, heart rate, pulse quality, skin turgor, mucous membrane color and moistness, capillary refill time (CRT), and blood pressure. Daily weighing of the patient should also be carried out at the same time each day to monitor overall fluid balance. Polyuria and polydipsia are common in these patients due to the effects of osmotic diuresis, so it is vital to quantitate urinary and other losses to ensure adequate fluid resuscitation.

Patients should be given the opportunity to urinate regularly, be kept clean, and provided with absorbent bedding. Urinary catheters with a closed collection system are ideal to quantify urinary losses, especially since these patients are often recumbent due to the neurologic effects of hyperosmolality. When a urinary catheter is in place, strict aseptic technique and efforts to control infection by diligent use of urinary catheter care protocols should be adhered to in order to prevent development of a urinary tract infection.

Neurologic assessment should be carried out frequently to assess the development, worsening, or resolution of clinical signs. Mentation, behavior, gait, posture, proprioception, and cranial nerve responses (including menace response, pupillary light reflex, and gag reflex) should also be assessed at regular intervals. Use of the Modified Glasgow Coma Scale can be beneficial for monitoring changes in neurologic status in these patients. The scale should be reassessed every 6–8 hr while neurologic signs are present.

Sodium levels should be monitored at intervals determined by the extent and severity of the derangement. Where the patient is showing clinical signs, this should be at least every 2 hr initially so that the rate of correction with fluid therapy treatment can be guided. Other electrolytes, including potassium, should also be monitored for changes and changes reported to the clinician so supplementation can be initiated when needed. Electrocardiogram (ECG) should be monitored if significant derangements in potassium are present. PCV/ TP and glucose should be regularly checked to ensure that hydration and hyper- glycemia (if diabetes or HHS is the underlying cause) are resolving. Placement of a central venous catheter or other sampling catheter is highly recommended for patient comfort due to the repeated sampling requirements needed. Minimum volume sampling should also be practiced to limit the development of iatrogenic anemia.

Plenty of padded bedding should be provided for patients with neurologic signs due to their recumbence and the potential for seizure activity. Anti-seizure medications such as diazepam should be administered as needed. If the patient is not ambulatory, they should have their position changed, or be turned, every 2–4 hr. Application of artificial tears every 2–4 hr may be required if the patient is in a comatose state.

Hypo-osmolar hyponatremia
Etiology
Hypo-osmolar hyponatremia is a true hyponatremia and can present with increased, decreased, or normal ECF volume. In order to determine the cause it is first necessary to establish the patient's volume status. This will then narrow the list of potential causes and guide further diagnostics.

Hypovolemic hyponatremia is seen when both sodium and fluid have been lost, with the loss of sodium being greater than that of water. Causes of fluid loss in this case can be defined as renal and non-renal. Non-renal losses include gastro- intestinal (GI) losses through vomiting and diarrhea, and third space losses (e.g. pleural effusion or peritoneal effusion, including uroabdomen and peritonitis). Hyponatremia due to vomiting and diarrhea develops not as a result of fluid loss itself, as this is usually hypotonic fluid loss, but as a result of the physiologic mechanisms to compensate for the volume depletion experienced. These mech- anisms work to preserve volume despite fluid tonicity and include:

1 GFR decreases in response to reduced renal blood flow. Reduced filtration rate leads to an increase in reabsorption of sodium and water in the proximal tubules of the kidneys, and reduced urinary output.
2 Baroreceptors in the aortic arch and carotid sinus respond to a reduction in circulating volume by stimulating the release of vasopressin from the posterior pituitary. This increases the reabsorption of water in the collecting duct and the DCT of the kidney.
3 Volume reduction also triggers the thirst response in the hypothalamus.

The net result of these mechanisms is the retention, or increased intake, of water and consequent dilution of sodium in the ECF. When a fluid deficit occurs due to third space losses, hypovolemic hyponatremia develops more simply as a result of the loss of sodium-rich fluid as an effusion or exudate.

The most common causes of renal sodium loss are through hypoadreno-corticism (Addison's disease) or diuretic administration (DiBartola 2012). Hypo-adrenocorticism results in a reduced or complete lack of production of mineralocorticoids, including aldosterone. In the absence of aldosterone, renal retention of sodium and water in the DCT and collecting ducts does not increase in response to the RAAS feedback system, so sodium is lost and the ECF volume becomes depleted. Volume depletion triggers protective mechanisms, including the thirst response, in order to maintain circulating volume, which further dilutes plasma sodium levels.

Diuretic administration can also lead to this state by enhancing loss of water in the renal tubules by inhibiting the reabsorption of sodium (and subsequently water). The extent of the effect from diuretics depends on a number of factors, including dose, clinical condition of the patient, and how early in renal tubule they take effect. Loop diuretics such as furosemide act in the LoH, thiazide diuretics such as hydrochlorothiazide act in the DCT, and potassium-sparing diuretics such as spironolactone act in the collecting duct. The efficacy of a particular class of diuretic is dependent on a number of factors, including dose, underlying disease process, and chronicity of treatment. Comparatively, however, loop diuretics exert the greatest effect on sodium by virtue of their site of action. In addition, vasopressin release and thirst response stimulated by volume depletion will cause further sodium dilution.

Hypervolemic hyponatremia is seen in three specific conditions:

- **Congestive heart failure (CHF):** Decreased cardiac output results in hypotension, which is detected as hypovolemia by baroreceptors, resulting in the release of vasopressin. Increased water reabsorption in the kidneys is augmented by the activation of the RAAS system in response to reduced renal perfusion. Despite sodium retention, hyponatremia is seen due to dilution of sodium with the greater increase in water retention and the lack of true initial hypovolemia.
- **Liver failure:** Ascites develops as a result of portal hypertension and decreased oncotic pressure resulting from hypoalbuminemia in liver failure. This in turn stimulates vasopressin release and activation of the RAAS system. Hyponatremia develops as a result of dilution with excess water retention.
- **Nephrotic syndrome:** Loss of excess proteins through an increase in permeability at the glomeruli leads to the development of hypoalbuminemia, edema, and subsequent decreased oncotic pressure. Activation of the RAAS system and vasopressin release leads to excess water retention and further sodium dilution.

In each case of hypervolemic hyponatremia, the sodium derangement occurs as a result of perceived volume deficit and initiation of physiologic mechanisms in an attempt to re-establish normovolemia. Normal renal water excretion is impaired and sodium is diluted. No matter the cause, deterioration will continue as a result of the inappropriate feedback mechanisms, thus prompt diagnosis and treatment of the underlying cause is essential to resolution in these patients.

Normovolemic hyponatremia is seen in patients with mild volume expansion due to continued vasopressin release or sustained excessive water intake. This leads to the development of natriuresis (urinary excretion of sodium) due to an increase in GFR and consequent inhibition of sodium and water reabsorption in the renal tubules. Causes include:

- **Psychogenic polydipsia:** This is a behavioral development that has been observed in dogs. It can occur in situations such as a learned behavior to gain attention, or as a displacement behavior in nervous or stressed animals (Nelson 2015).
- **SIADH:** Syndrome of inappropriate anti-diuretic hormone secretion is seen when vasopressin is released inappropriately in the absence of volume depletion or increased plasma osmolality. SIADH is rare in dogs (Mazzaferro 2013).
- **Administration of hypotonic fluids:** Iatrogenic hyponatremia can be seen through the administration of hypotonic fluids as routine fluid therapy in patients with impaired water excretion. Impaired water excretion can be seen where patients have increase stimuli or vasopressin release such as sick or hospitalized patients experiencing postoperative pain, stress, and anxiety (Bagshaw Townsend, & McDermid 2009).
- **Administration of drugs with antidiuretic effects:** These include drugs such as barbiturates, narcotics, and chlorpropamide that stimulate the release of, or potentiate the effects of, vasopressin. Vincristine and cyclophosphamide also impair water excretion (DiBartola 2012).
- **Myxedema coma:** is a rare complication of untreated, chronic severe hypothyroidism or an acute hypothyroid crisis impacts a number of organ systems. Exact mechanisms are not known, but there are a few reasons proposed for hyponatremia in these patients, including increased vasopressin release and reduced aldosterone release (Hess 2009).

Clinical signs

The rate of onset and magnitude of the derangement are the most significant factors when considering clinical signs. As plasma sodium levels reduce, water moves into the ICF in response to changes in the osmotic gradient. This includes movement of water into the brain cells, causing them to swell. In chronic cases, the brain protects itself from cellular swelling by mirroring the osmolality of the ECF. This is achieved through the efflux of organic osmolytes such as taurine, glycine, and myo-inositol from the cells and occurs over a period of around two days. In acute cases, however, where the rate of sodium reduction exceeds 0.5 mEq/L/hr, or drops to less than 120 mEq/L, this protective mechanism cannot keep up with the change. Consequently, the brain cells swell with the influx of water and in an enclosed space and increased intracranial pressure develops. At worst brain herniation and death may occur. Clinical signs may be seen as mild at first including lethargy, nausea, and slight weight gain, progressing to vomiting, discernible weight gain, and eventually coma.

Treatment

As with all sodium derangements, treatment varies as it must be directed at the underlying cause. In chronic or mild cases where clinical signs related to hyponatremia are absent, it may not be necessary to correct sodium levels. In fact, there is potential in these cases to do further harm to the patient through initiation of aggressive treatment. When sodium levels have fallen over a period of 48 hr, brain cells instigate adaptive mechanisms to match the reducing osmolality of the ECF. Rapid correction of sodium therefore may lead to complications in the form of osmotic demyelination syndrome (ODS) (King & Rosner 2010). Demyelination refers to damage of the protective myelin sheath that surrounds nerve fibers, and occurs when the brain does not have time to resynthesize the osmolytes it has lost to keep up with the increasing osmolality of the ECF. Water moves out of the brain cells, leading to cellular damage, which leads to disruption of the blood–brain barrier. This in turn permits entry of inflammatory mediators to the CNS, which may damage and ultimately cause demyelination of nerve cells. Clinical signs of ODS develop over a period of 3–4 days and may include lethargy, weakness, ataxia, dysphagia, loss of postural and proprioceptive responses, decreased menace response, hypermetria, and quadriparesis (King & Rosner 2010).

In addition to treating the underlying cause, treatment focused on returning sodium levels to normal may be required in some patients (Table 2.2). Patients that are asymptomatic require minimal treatment, but water intake should be restricted and closely monitored. Sodium levels should be regularly checked to establish that they are gradually returning to normal and patients observed closely to ensure the continued absence of clinical signs. Symptomatic patients should be treated with an isotonic crystalloid fluid with sodium content closest to the current plasma sodium of the patient. The aim is to increase sodium levels at a rate no greater than 0.5 mEq/L/hr or 10–12 mEq/L/day. The patient's volume status must also be considered and the use or restriction of diuretics instituted as necessary (Table 2.2).

Nursing care and monitoring

In addition to the general monitoring of hydration and neurologic status discussed in the nursing care of hyperosmolar hyponatremia, fluid intake should be quantitated and recorded, possibly being restricted when necessary. Urine output should be closely monitored and recorded in order to aid volume and overall hydration assessment. In addition, more focused monitoring of volume status is required, as treatment will in part be aimed at addressing

Table 2.2 Treatment recommendations for hyponatremia based on clinical signs (Source: Data adapted from DiBartola 2012)

	Hypovolemic	Normovolemic	Hypervolemic
Asymptomatic	Replacement of water deficit with isotonic fluid (e.g. 0.9% NaCl, LRS) Mild water restriction and monitoring of sodium levels	Water intake restricted to less than urine output Discontinuation of drugs known to precipitate hyponatremia where possible Monitoring of sodium levels	Dietary sodium restriction in edematous patients Mild water restriction and monitoring of sodium levels
Symptomatic	Initiation of IVF therapy using crystalloids (0.9% NaCl or LRS) Increase sodium at rates not exceeding 0.5 mEq/L/ hr or 10–12 mEq/L/day	Initiation of IVF therapy using crystalloids (0.9% NaCl or LRS) Increase sodium at rates not exceeding 0.5 mEq/L/hr or 10–12 mEq/L/day	Administration of loop diuretics with concurrent administration of 0.9% NaCl Increase sodium at rates not exceeding 0.5 mEq/L/ hr or 10–12 mEq/L/day

LRS: Lactated Ringer's solution.

volume discrepancies. Patients suffering from CHF may require a sodium-restricted diet, depending on the extent of their underlying disease.

All patients should be closely monitored for signs of volume overload to prevent overcorrection of hypovolemia or exacerbation of existing hypervolemia. These signs may include pulmonary crackles, increased blood pressure, increased central venous pressure, increased urine output, jugular venous distension, widened pulse pressure, dyspnea, tachycardia, and peripheral edema. Chest radiographs may be required to evaluate the presence and extent of pulmonary edema if present.

Signs of volume deficit may also be observed in response to overzealous treatment of hypervolemia or presenting hypovolemia. Signs include oliguria (urine output of less than 0.5 mL/kg/hour), poor skin turgor, tachycardia, weak, narrow pulse, and hypotension. Development or deterioration of neurologic status, hyper- or hypovolemia, and rapid changes in blood parameters should be brought to the attention of the clinician immediately.

Hypernatremia

Hypernatremia reportedly occurs much less commonly than hyponatremia and describes plasma sodium levels greater than 160 mEq/L (Nelson, Delaney, & Elliot 2009). In a normal patient, development of hypernatremia is typically prevented by the normal protective physiologic mechanisms of the body, which include release of vasopressin and the thirst response. In the clinical setting, hypernatremia can be broken down into three categories: normovolemic, hypo-volemic, and hypervolemic.

Etiology

Normovolemic hypernatremia occurs as a result of a "free water deficit," or loss of pure water from the ECF. It is seen when an animal has no access to water (e.g. a cat shut in a garage when the owners are away on vacation with no access to water, or a frozen water bowl), or when an animal is suffering from primary hypodipsia (e.g. due to neoplasia or trauma affecting the thirst center of the hypothalamus resulting in a lack of thirst recognition). Diabetes insipidus (DI) can also cause hypernatremia through increased water loss from inadequate release of vasopressin (central or pituitary DI) or lack of response to vasopressin in the kidney (nephrogenic DI). This results in loss of pure water, which causes the ECF to become hypertonic in relation to the ICF (i.e. a greater concentration of osmoles per volume of water). Water subsequently moves from the ICF to the ECF to create equilibrium, resulting in proportional volume loss between compartments.

Hypovolemic hypernatremia is caused by the loss of "hypotonic fluid," or fluid containing fewer solutes than the fluid within the ECF. Causes of hypotonic fluid loss break down into extra-renal and renal fluid losses. The most common cause of extra-renal loss is from the GI tract, due to vomiting and diarrhea. Less commonly this type of loss may occur due to third spacing, as in cases of peritonitis, or cutaneous losses from severe burns. Renal losses may also occur if there is an inability to concentrate urine (e.g. in chronic renal failure, non-oliguric acute renal failure, post-obstructive diuresis, and drug administration including genta-mycin, amphotericin B, methoxyflurane) or may also be due to diuresis (either drug induced, e.g. furosemide or corticosteroids, or osmotic, e.g. ketonurina, glucosuria, or mannitol administration; DiBartola 2012). In comparison to pure water loss, hypotonic fluid loss stimulates a less dramatic fluid shifting from the ICF to the ECF in order to re-establish equilibrium. As a result, these patients frequently present with a degree of hypovolemia.

Hypervolemic hypernatremia is the least common cause of hypernatremia in veterinary medicine and is seen when sodium, or other impermeant solutes, is gained (Mazzaferro 2013). Causes include excess salt ingestion (e.g. ingestion of homemade salt, playdough, or the use of salt as an emetic) or the addition of an alternate impermeant solute—such as mannitol, glucose, or sodium bicarbo-nate—to the ECF. Hyperaldosteronism and hyperadrenocorticism have also been linked with hypervolemic hypernatremia (Kochevar & Scott 2013). In these patients, the high levels of sodium or impermeant solute causes an overall increase in solute concentration, or osmolarity, in the ECF. This causes water to shift from the ICF and interstitial fluids (ISF) spaces into the ECF.

Mild hyponatremia may initially be seen in cases where the addition of glucose or mannitol to plasma creates a hyperosmolar hyponatremia, as described previously. Calculating corrected sodium in the cases with hyperglycemia will uncover some of these occult cases. Following this initial stage, osmotic diuresis begins in these patients because the impermeant solute pulls water with it as it is excreted in the urine. The impermeant solute being excreted is done in exchange for sodium, causing sodium retention and hypernatremia develops.

Clinical signs

The clinical signs of hypernatremia depend on the severity and how quickly it developed. Neurologic signs occur as water moves out of the brain cells as a result of the increased sodium concentration, or osmolality, of the ECF. In cats and dogs, neurologic signs are generally not seen until plasma sodium exceeds 170 mEq/L (Hardy 1989).

In acute cases of hypernatremia, neurologic signs develop as a result of dehydration of brain cells. Signs may include anorexia, lethargy, vomiting, muscular weakness, disorientation, ataxia, seizures, coma, and death. If the dehydration is severe, ruptured blood vessels and focal hemorrhage may also occur (Nelson, Delaney, & Elliot 2009; DiBartola 2012). If hypotonic fluid loss is the cause, signs of volume depletion are often seen, including tachycardia, weak pulses, and prolonged capillary refill time. Conversely, if solute gain is the cause, signs of volume overload may be found, including bounding pulses, increased respiratory rate, and pulmonary crackles may be auscultated. Patients with existing cardiac disease are especially prone to developing pulmonary edema secondary to the hypervolemia.

In chronic cases of hypernatremia, neurologic signs are often less evident due to the brain's production of idiogenic osmoles or osmolytes. These are organic osmoles produced to protect the brain cells from becoming dehydrated due to the hyperosmolality in the ECF. Production is thought to begin within a few hours of the initial increase in ECF and continues until the osmolality of brain cells matches that of the ECF. This helps prevent water loss and subsequent cell dehydration (Kochevar & Scott 2013).

Treatment

The treatment of hypernatremia poses a number of complications, as the degree of hypernatremia, the patient's volume status, as well as the length of time that the hypernatremia has been present must all be considered. If the imbalance has occurred over a prolonged, or unknown, period of time (>24–48 hr), idiogenic osmoles will have been produced in sufficient number to protect the brain tissue from dehydration (King & Rosner 2010). Consequently, rapid correction of hypernatremia will result in lowering the osmolality of the ECF to less than the osmolality of the ICF in the brain. This will cause an influx of fluid into the ICF, causing cerebral edema to occur. Correction of chronic hypernatremia should therefore be carried out gradually over a minimum of 48–72 hr to allow for the dissipation of these solutes and normalization of fluid balance between the ICF in the brain and the ECF of the body.

The primary focus for treatment is to correct the volume deficit, if present, and identify and treat the underlying cause. In most cases of hypernatremia, an isotonic solution such as 0.9% NaCl should be selected for initial volume replacement (DiBartola 2012). In cases of severe chronic hypernatremia, fluid sodium levels may need to be adjusted to closer match the patient's current sodium level during the rehydration period. This is in order to limit the chances of inducing rapid changes in plasma sodium levels through the administration of isotonic fluids with an osmolality, or sodium level, significantly lower than the current plasma level. This can be calculated using the following equation:

Patient's Na^+ − Na^+ in fluid = Na^+ to add to 1 L of fluid

The addition of hypertonic saline to a 0.9% solution may be considered to bring up the fluid's sodium levels as needed. The fluid type selected should be continually adjusted based on the patient's current plasma sodium levels throughout treatment, until normalized. If the length of time the patient has been hypernatremic is unknown, it should be assumed chronic until proven otherwise, and treated as such.

In known acute cases rapid correction may be tolerated. However, in the majority of cases, the development period will be unknown, therefore gradual correction over a period of 48 hr is still often the best approach (Burton & Theodore 2001). Regular monitoring of the sodium levels must be carried out to ensure that the rate of correction does not exceed 0.5 mEq/L/hr, or 12 mEq/L/24 hr.

In patients with pure water or hypotonic water loss, the water deficit should be calculated using the following equation (Kochevar & Scott 2013):

$$\text{Water deficit }(L)=0.6\times\text{total bodyweight }(kg)\times\left[\left(\text{patient's }Na^+/\text{normal }Na^+\right)-1\right]$$

Water deficits should be replaced over the time it takes to normalize sodium levels (48–72 hr minimally in most cases).

In cases of hypervolemic hypernatremia, the above protocol should still be followed, with judicious fluid administration and close monitoring for signs of volume overload (bounding pulses, increased respiratory rate, and crackles on auscultation). Patients with normal cardiac and renal function will excrete the excess sodium and water in the urine through natriuresis and diuresis. In patients that develop, or are at risk of developing, pulmonary edema as a result of underlying cardiac or renal disease, the use of diuretics such as furosemide will assist in volume reduction.

In addition to IVF therapy in hypernatremic patients, if no vomiting or diarrhea is present, placement of a nasoesophageal or nasogastric tube may be considered to administer a slow constant rate infusion (CRI) of water. The GI tract will not absorb water at a rate that will lower plasma sodium too fast for that particular patient. So this can be a useful adjunctive treatment method, especially in patients whose hypernatremia is not resolving adequately with IV fluids alone (i.e. sodium levels are coming down at less than 10 mEq/day).

Nursing care/Monitoring

Nursing care of the hypernatremic patient is aimed at evaluating the patient's response to treatment and keeping the clinician informed of changes to achieve steady improvement and prevent further deterioration in clinical condition.

Volume and hydration status should be closely monitored for signs of deterioration or overcorrection. Heart rate, respiratory rate and effort, pulse quality, skin turgor, mucous membrane color and moistness, CRT, and blood pressure should be regularly assessed. The patient should be weighed daily to assess overall fluid balance, and any notable increases or losses reported to the clinician. Osmotic diuresis may occur as a result of the underlying cause or in response to initiation of treatment. Patients with diarrhea should be kept clean to prevent scalding of their skin around the rectum and may therefore require frequent walks and bedding checks. Bedding should be well padded to minimize self-trauma in patients with neurologic signs and seizures. Anti-seizure medications should be administered if needed. Patients with muscular weakness may require support to mobilize the patient as well as frequent turning if recumbent. Placement of a urinary catheter should be considered to minimize the risk of urinary scalding in recumbent patients and to closely monitor losses.

The patient's neurologic status should be assessed frequently during the course of corrective treatment with the goal of resolving existing, or preventing the onset of, clinical signs. The Modified Glasgow Coma Scale or similar objective tools should be used to assess level of consciousness (LOC). Mentation, behavior, gait, posture, proprioception, and cranial nerve responses (including menace response, pupillary light reflex, and gag reflex) should be assessed at regular intervals.

The patient should be observed for signs of nausea (including salivation, swallowing, and lip licking). Use of anti-emetics may be required. Eating may need to be encouraged in animals that are anorectic. In patients that have had a lack of access to water, reintroduction of water should be gradual and intake and urine output should be carefully monitored and quantified.

Frequent assessment of plasma sodium should be conducted along with packed cell volume (PCV) and total protein (TP) to monitor the response to hydration and volume replacement efforts. In severe or acute cases where clinical signs are observed, sodium should be checked at least every 2 hr initially to ensure that the rate of correction is not exceeding 0.5 mEq/L/hr. Changes in plasma sodium should be brought to the attention of the clinician, as this will guide adjustments to the sodium concentration of the fluid therapy. Other electrolytes, including potassium, should also be monitored for imbalances and treated accordingly. ECG monitoring should be considered if potassium is significantly altered.

Placement of a central venous catheter or alternative sampling catheter should be considered for patient comfort and due to the likely length of hospitalization, required to treat this electrolyte derangement. Minimum volume sampling should also be practiced where possible to avoid the development of iatrogenic anemia. The clinician should be alerted to changes or deterioration in any of the above.

References

Bagshaw, S. M., Townsend, D. R., & McDermid, R. C. (2009). Disorders of sodium and water balance in hospitalized patients. *Canadian Journal of Anaesthesia* **56**(2): 151–67.

Bohn, A. A. (2012). Laboratory evaluation of electrolytes. In: M. A. Thrall, G. Weiser, R. Allison, & T. Campbell (eds), *Veterinary Hematology and Clinical Chemistry*. Oxford: Wiley-Blackwell: 378–400.

Burton, D. R. & Theodore, W. P. (2001). *Clinical Physiology of Acid-Base and Electrolyte Disorders*. New York: McGraw-Hill.

DiBartola, S. P. (2012). Disorders of sodium and water: Hypernatremia and hyponatremia. In: S. P. DiBartola (ed.), *Fluid, Electrolyte, and Acid-Base Disorders in Small Animal Practice*. St Louis, MO: Elsevier Saunders: 80–91.

Guyton, A. C. & Hall, J. E. (2011). *Guyton and Hall Textbook of Medical Physiology*. St Louis, MO: Saunders Elsevier.

Hardy, R. M. (1989). Hypernatremia. *Veterinary Clinics of North America Small Animal Practice* **19**(2): 231–40.

Hess, R. S. (2009). Myxedema coma. In: D. C. Silverstein & K. Hopper (eds), *Small Animal Critical Care Medicine*. St Louis, MO: Saunders Elsevier: 311–313.

Hillier, T. A., Abbott, R. D., & Barrett, E. J. (1999). Hyponatremia: Evaluating the correction factor for hyperglycemia. *American Journal of Medicine* **106**(4): 399–403.

King, J. D. & Rosner, M. H. (2010). Osmotic demyelination syndrome. *American Journal of the Medical Sciences* **339**(6): 561–7.

Kochevar, D. T. & Scott, M. M. (2013). Principles of acid-base balance: Fluid and electrolyte therapy. In: J. E. Riviere & M. G. Papich (eds), *Veterinary Pharmacology and Therapeutics*. Ames, IA: Wiley-Blackwell: 605–46.

Koenig, A. (2009). Hyperglycemic hyperosmolar syndrome. In: D. C. Silverstein & K. Hopper (eds), *Small Animal Critical Care Medicine*. St Louis, MO: Saunders Elsevier: 291–4.

Mazzaferro, E. M. (2013). *Small Animal Fluid Therapy, Acid-Base and Electrolyte Disorders*. London: Manson Publishing.

Nelson, R. W. (2015). Water metabolism and diabetes insipidus. In: E. C. Feldman, R. W. Nelson, C. Reusch, et al. (eds), *Canine and Feline Endocrinology*. St Louis, MO: Elsevier Saunders: 1–36.

Nelson, R. W., Delaney, S. J., & Elliot D. A. (2009). Electrolyte imbalances. In: R. W. Nelson & C. G. Couto (eds), *Small Animal Internal Medicine*. St Louis, MO: Mosby Elsevier: 864–83.

Robertson, G. L. (1983). Thirst and vasopressin function in normal and disordered states of water balance. *Journal of Laboratory and Clinical Medicine* **101**(3): 351–71.

Schricker, K., Hamann, M., & Kurtz, A. (1995). Nitric oxide and prostaglandins are involved in the macula densa control of the renin system. *American Journal of Physiology* **269**: 825–30.

Stephenson, R. B. (2007). Neural and hormonal control of blood pressure and blood volume. In: J. G. Cunningham & B. G. Kelin (eds), *Textbook of Veterinary Physiology*. St Louis, MO: Elsevier Saunders: 276–85.

Wellman, M. L., DiBartola, S. P., & Kohn, C. W. (2012). Applied physiology of body fluids in dogs and cats. In: S. P. DiBartola (ed.), *Fluid, Electrolyte, and Acid-Base Disorders in Small Animal Practice*. St Louis, MO: Elsevier Saunders: 2–25.

CHAPTER 3

Disorders of Chloride

Meri Hall, RVT, LVT, CVT, LATG, VTS (SAIM)

Chloride (Cl⁻), like all electrolytes, is distributed in the intracellular fluid (ICF), interstitial fluid (ISF), and extracellular fluid (ECF) spaces. Chloride is the strongest of the major anions in the mammalian body. It is the primary anion in ECF with the majority of it found in the plasma, accounting for approximately two-thirds of all anions in the ECF. Normal plasma concentrations of chloride are 110–120 mEq/L in canines and felines, respectively. Intracellular levels of chloride are lower and vary in concentration depending on the cellular resting membrane potential. For example, the chloride concentrations in muscle cells are 2–4 mEq/L and in the red blood cells they are 60 mEq/L (DiBartola 2012). Because nature wants to maintain electroneutrality, chloride usually is found paired with a positively charged anion. The two major positively charged ions in the body fluids are sodium (Na^+) and potassium (K^+). The positive charges of sodium and potassium create a balance with the negative charge of chloride to maintain serum osmolarity and to conduct electrical impulses within the body.

Chloride homeostasis in the body is maintained by chloride transporters that actively transport chloride across the cellular membrane by way of chloride channels. These chloride channels are anion selective and found in intracellular organelles and the plasma membrane. They assist in the regulation of skeletal, smooth and cardiac muscle, transepithelial salt transport, cell cycle, regulation of the excitability of neurons, and acidification of extracellular and intracellular fluids. The movement of chloride into the cell via active transport through chloride channels promotes the nervous electrical potential. If the chloride transporters are altered due to mutation or dysfunction hyperexcitability or hypoexcitability of the nervous system can be the result. In the body, all halides use the same receptors, so another halide may replace or compete with chloride on the chloride channel. Dysfunction or swelling of chloride transporters has been shown to cause secondary effects of cerebral edema after traumatic and

Acid-Base and Electrolyte Handbook for Veterinary Technicians, First Edition.
Edited by Angela Randels-Thorp and David Liss.
© 2017 John Wiley & Sons, Inc. Published 2017 by John Wiley & Sons, Inc.
Companion website: www.wiley.com/go/liss/electrolytes

ischemic brain injury. The strength and polarity of gamma-amino butyric acid (GABA) mediated neurotransmission is dependent on the intracellular chloride concentration (DiBartola 2012).

Chloride is involved with maintaining the homeostasis of volume, the transportation of organic solutes, and plays an important role in the acid-base balance by the regulation of pH (discussed further in Chapter 11). An inverse relationship exists within the body between chloride and bicarbonate (HCO_3^-). When there is a decrease in chloride, there is a relative increase in bicarbonate.

Physiology of chloride

Chloride is an essential mineral in the diet of animals. Chloride is found in most pet foods produced today. Whole grains, meats, and fish provide the essential chloride to the diet. Many commercially produced pet foods are supplemented with sodium chloride, so deficiencies are rare. The chloride in the diet is approximately 91–99% bioavailable and is absorbed by active or passive transport across the gastrointestinal (GI) wall by the electrical gradient that is produced with sodium transport. Once absorbed, chloride is utilized by the body to assist with the metabolism of other nutrients.

In the stomach, chloride combines with hydrogen (H^+) to form hydrochloric acid. The hydrochloric acid along with pepsinogen begins breaking down the food so it can be digested and the individual nutrients can be absorbed by the body. As the ingesta travels into the jejunum, where chloride is transported through the gastric lumen following sodium and is exchanged for bicarbonate (HCO_3^-) to maintain electrical neutrality across the membrane. This reabsorbed chloride is returned to the bloodstream, where it maintains the ECF volume. Dependent on the metabolic demands chloride is actively and passively absorbed. Homeostasis is maintained by the constant exchange of bicarbonate and chloride between the plasma and red blood cells to govern the pH balance. As the material flows through the GI tract, further absorption occurs. In the ileum bicarbonate is secreted and more chloride is absorbed. The secretion and absorption is due to the active transport of either bicarbonate, chloride, or both. The colon is highly efficient in the absorption of chloride and up to 90% of the chloride in the fecal material is absorbed. As fecal material reaches the distal colon, active chloride resorption continues with secretion of bicarbonate. Therefore, animals with vomiting or diarrhea can lose large amounts of chloride which can create metabolic alkalosis.

The kidneys play an important role in the regulation of chloride within the body. Chloride is the predominant anion in the glomerular filtrate and 80% of the reabsorbed sodium is accompanied by chloride. Within the renal tubules, chloride is filtered and reabsorbed by both passive and active transport systems. Approximately 50–60% of chloride is absorbed in the proximal convoluted and straight tubules, and transcellulary within the ascending limb of the loop of Henle. Medications can disrupt the reabsorption of chloride within the body. Patients who are on diuretic therapy may lose chloride in the urine. Because diuretics compete for or block the chloride receptors, the chloride reabsorption does not occur. Loop diuretics such as furosemide promote diuresis in the loop of Henle by competing for the chloride site on Na^+–K^+–$2Cl^-$ carriers. Another type of diuretic, thiazide diuretics, inhibit the NaCl carrier in the distal tubule, and the NaCl is excreted in the urine. For patients with seizure disorders, who are on potassium bromide therapy (KBr), bromide (Br^-) competes with chloride at the chloride receptors in the renal tubules which also affect resorption or excretion rates.

Measurement

Chloride can be measured in serum, plasma, blood, cerebrospinal fluid, and urine. Serum is the preferred sample because the chloride ion is stable for months. In small animal veterinary medicine, the urine chloride is seldom measured, because it typically correlates to sodium excretion. In human medicine, urine chloride is measured to diagnose dehydration and monitor the fluid and electrolyte balance in postoperative patients. In veterinary patients, alkaline urine is often a result of excretion of sodium bicarbonate. Therefore measurement of urine chloride levels may be beneficial to provide evidence of volume contraction (Creedon & Davis 2012).

Older chemistry assays were unable to distinguish between various types of halides and any halide was reported as chloride. This posed a problem, especially for patients receiving potassium bromide therapy for seizure disorders as these units would potentially report a false increase in chloride readings. The newer analyzers, so long as they are not electrode analyzers, do not have this problem anymore. In samples that are lipemic or hyperproteinemic, however, chloride levels can be reported artificially low with current biochemistry machines. This is not a true hypochloremia but rather what is termed pseudohypochloremia.

The average plasma concentration in dogs is 110 mEq/L and 120 mEq/L in cats (DiBartola 2012). The levels in venous blood are 3–4 mEq/L lower than arterial samples, and in cerebrospinal fluid the levels are 15–20 mEq/L higher than serum (Irani 2008).

Evaluation

There are generally no clinical signs associated with derangements in chloride levels alone. The clinical signs seen are typically associated with the concurrent disease process or acid-base abnormality that may exist in that patient. Chloride is evaluated as part of the strong ion difference and plays a major role in the metabolic component of acid-base regulations (See Chapter 11). When evaluating chloride levels they should always be evaluated in conjunction with sodium levels. Sodium and chloride should exist at a ratio of 3:2. The average normal

$$Cl^- [corrected] = Cl^- [measured] \times \frac{Na^+ [normal]}{Na^+ [measured]}$$

$$\text{Dogs: } Cl^- [corrected] = Cl^- \times \frac{146 \text{ mEq/L}}{Na^+ [measured]}$$

$$\text{Cats: } Cl^- [corrected] = Cl^- \times \frac{156 \text{ mEq/L}}{Na^+ [measured]}$$

Figure 3.1 Corrected chloride.

$$\text{Chloride gap} = Cl^- [normal] - Cl^- [corrected]$$

$$\text{Dogs: } (110 \text{ mEq/L} - [measured]) \, Cl^- \text{ of the patient} \times \frac{146 \text{ mEq/L}}{Na^+ [measured]}$$

$$\text{Cats: } (120 \text{ mEq/L} - [measured]) \, Cl^- \text{ of the patient} \times \frac{156 \text{ mEq/L}}{Na^+ [measured]}$$

Figure 3.2 Chloride gap.

level of sodium is approximately 146 mEq/L in dogs, and 156 mEq/L in cats. The normal chloride value is 105–115 mEq/L in dogs and 115–125 mEq/L in cats (DiBartola 2012).

Disorders of chloride can be divided into either artifactual or true derangements and must be evaluated in relation to changes of sodium and water balance. To obtain a more accurate picture, the chloride value must also be corrected. If the change is due to free water, the changes of sodium and chloride are proportional. The corrected chloride value is obtained using the formula in Figure 3.1. The values used for normal sodium levels in this formula are 146 mEq/L and 156 mEq/L for canines and felines respectively. The normal range for corrected chloride values in dogs is 107–113 mEq/L and for cats is 117–123 mEq/L. If the corrected chloride is normal then the change is artifactual. If the corrected chloride is abnormal then the abnormality detected is true.

The chloride gap (Figure 3.2) is the average normal chloride value subtracting the measured corrected chloride value. The numbers for the average normal chloride value for dogs is 110 mEq/L and for cats is 120 mEq/L and should be used in this calculation. For both species, if the chloride gap is more than 4 mEq/L, the patient is in hypochloremic alkalosis. If the chloride gap is less than 4 mEq/L, the patient is in hyperchloremic acidosis.

$$\text{Ratio} = \frac{Cl^-}{Na^+}$$

Figure 3.3 Sodium chloride ratio.

Another quick estimate of the chloride status would be a chloride:sodium ratio (Figure 3.3). The ratio is easily obtained with chemistry results. If the ratio is greater than 0.78 in dogs or greater than 0.80 in cats, the patient is in hyperchloremic acidosis. If the ratio is less than 0.72 for dogs and 0.74 for cats, the patient is in hypochloremic alkalosis.

The sodium-to-chloride difference can also be calculated to evaluate if the chloride derangement is true. If the sodium is normal, the difference is approximately 36 mEq/L. If the sodium is normal and the difference is greater than 40 mEq/L, there is a hypochloremic alkalosis, and if less than 32 mEq/L, a hyperchloremic acidosis is present.

Hyperchloremia

Increases in the chloride levels are often found in patients with metabolic acidosis. There is usually a normal anion gap and a decrease in the plasma bicarbonate concentration. In some cases, patients may have a pseudohyperchloremia due to potassium bromide administration (if electrode modalities are used), hemoglobinemia, lipemia, or bilirubinemia. Additionally, colorimetric assays cannot distinguish between hemoglobin and bilirubin and falsely high readings may result.

Causes of hyperchloremia

Hyperchloremia may be artifactual, due to disease, iatrogenic, or dietary causes (Box 3.1). Artifactual changes are due to changes in free water. In these patients the mean chloride reading will be high, but the corrected chloride calculation will be normal. These changes are typically due to a disease causing free water loss, such as diabetes insipidus; or a hypotonic fluid loss, from an osmotic diuresis; or a sodium gain, from either an iatrogenic cause, or hyperadrenocorticism. These patients lean towards developing metabolic alkalosis. This fact aids in differentiating an artifactual hyperchloremic patient from one with a corrected hyperchloremia, as a patient with corrected hyperchloremia would lean towards developing an acidosis.

Pseudohyperchloremia may also occur. Depending on laboratory equipment used to measure chloride levels, pseudohypochloremic results may occur in patients with lipemic or hyperproteinemic samples. Machines that utilize titrimetric methods to measure chloride will underestimate chloride values if triglyceride concentrations are >600 mg/dL. These patients are not actually hypochloremic: it is laboratory error.

Box 3.1 Causes of hyperchloremia (Source: Based on data from Mazzaferro 2013)

Artifactual

Bilirubinemia
Diabetes insipidus
Hemoglobinemia
Lipemia
Osmotic diuresis
Potassium bromide

True

Disease processes
- Chronic respiratory alkalosis
- Diabetes mellitus
- Renal failure
- Renal tubular acidosis

Drug administration
- Acetazolamide
- Potassium sparing diuretics
  - amiloride
  - spironolactone

Intravenous fluids
- 0.9% NaCl
- Hypertonic saline
- Potassium chloride
- Magnesium chloride

Parenteral nutrition

A variety of disease processes may result in a "true" corrected hyperchloremia. Pseudohyperchloremia should be ruled out. Once it is, and the corrected chloride confirms hyperchloremia, then the derangement may be considered true. Kidney disease or failure may result in renal retention of chloride, resulting in a true corrected hyperchloremia. Many patients who present with prolonged diarrhea are hyperchloremic due to the loss of bicarbonate and excessive loss of sodium compared to loss of chloride and fluids (DiBartola 2012). Diabetes mellitus with ketones, or diabetic ketoacidotic (DKA) patients, will also develop corrected hyperchloremia due to the kidneys excreting keto acids instead of chloride, thereby increasing the chloride concentration in the plasma and developing a metabolic acidosis. DKA patients may present with or develop this electrolyte disturbance during resolution of the DKA crisis. Utilization of 0.9% NaCl, especially with supplementation of potassium chloride (KCl), will often result in a corrected hyperchloremic state. If large amounts of 0.9% NaCl with supplemental KCl are used in a DKA patient, they are doubly predisposed to developing corrected hyperchloremia, subsequently worsening their metabolic acidosis. Other diseases—like hypoadrenocorticism, chronic respiratory alkalosis, or renal tubular acidosis—may also cause this electrolyte disturbance.

Fluid therapy to replace losses or fluid deficits in veterinary patients may result in an iatrogenic hyperchloremia due to administration of saline and KCl supplementation. Care must be taken when administering chloride-containing fluids during rehydration or when using hypertonic saline during resuscitation efforts on patients with severe hypovolemia, as an increase in the blood sodium levels will also increase the blood chloride levels. Iatrogenic hyperchloremia may also be seen in patients with osmotic diuresis. Administration of certain drugs may also promote chloride retention and loss of bicarbonate. Potassium-sparing diuretics, such as spironolactone, inhibit sodium reabsorption and chloride is retained. Acetazolamide has been shown to result in the loss of bicarbonate in the urine and chloride retention in the kidneys.

Animals do not usually have increased dietary chloride intake, but some diets for management of crystalluria or with increased salt levels may attribute to hyperchloremia. Administration of parenteral nutrition may result in hyperchloremia if care is not taken to balance the formulas to account for disease processes and intravenous fluid administration.

Clinical signs

Clinical signs of hyperchloremia are the same as for patients with metabolic acidosis and depend on the underlying disease status of the patient. There are no specific clinical signs associated with hyperchloremia, but rather are associated with metabolic acidosis or are nonspecific, such as: Kussmaul respirations, polydipsia, weakness, lethargy, tachypnea, polyuria, hypertension, hypernatremia, and hyposthenuria. If left untreated, patients with severe metabolic acidosis (pH < 7.2) may experience dysrhythmias that could result in decreased cardiac output (Feldman & Nelson 2004; Mazzaferro 2013).

Treatment

Treatment of hyperchloremia includes the correction of the underlying disease, fluid therapy, and possibly administration of bicarbonate if the pH is < 7.2 (Feldman & Nelson 2004; Mazzaferro 2013). Care must be taken to administer fluids that are balanced to prevent exacerbation of the existing hyperchloremia, especially in patients receiving prolonged administration of 0.9% saline and KCl. Patients with diabetes mellitus, DKA, or any degree of renal compromise should be given extra consideration due to their predisposition of developing corrected hyperchloremia during hospitalization and fluid therapy, even if normal at presentation.

Hypochloremia

Artificial changes in a patient's chloride levels causing them to appear hypochloremic may occur when there is a change in free water. No true imbalance of electrolytes actually exists in these cases. Parallel changes of both sodium and chloride will be seen in these patients. Hypochloremia represents a low chloride level. In a patient with artifactual hypochloremia, however, when the corrected chloride is calculated, it is found to be within the normal range. That the patient's corrected chloride is normal does not mean there is no clinical significance to these results, however. Artifactual hypochloremia can be associated with, though not pathognomonic for, specific diseases or processes such as hypoadrenocorticism, congestive heart failure, and third space losses, as well as some GI losses if the patient is experiencing both vomiting and diarrhea. Also of note, patients with artificial hypochloremia are predisposed to acidosis, whereas a patient with a true corrected hypochloremia would experience an alkalosis.

Depending on laboratory equipment used to measure chloride levels, pseudohypochloremic results may occur in patients with lipemic or hyperproteinemic samples. Machines that utilize titrimetric methods to measure chloride will underestimate chloride values if triglyceride concentrations are >600 mg/dL. These patients are not actually hypochloremic: it is laboratory error.

True hypochloremic patients have a decrease in the number of chloride ions, which results in a metabolic alkalosis. Corrected hypochloremia, after confirming by the formula for corrected chloride, will show a decrease in chloride with a likelihood of alkalosis. If pseudohypochloremia has been ruled out then a cause for the hypochloremia should be sought. These patients may have an excess of bicarbonate, administration of something containing more sodium than chloride (compared to ECF), or an increase in the loss of chloride from the body. Hypochloremic metabolic alkalosis can be further differentiated between chloride responsive or chloride resistant. If metabolic alkalosis corrects with treatment involving intravenous administration of 0.9% NaCl or fluids containing KCl, it is Cl⁻ responsive. If the patient's hypochloremic metabolic alkalosis does not correct with chloride administration, it is termed chloride resistant. Patients with hypochloremia frequently have concurrent hypokalemia additionally.

Causes of hypochloremia

Hypochloremia rarely is observed in the absence of other abnormalities (Box 3.2). A decrease in chloride can be seen in patients with vomiting, use of loop diuretics, hyperadrenocorticism (Cushing's disease) and post steroid administration. Chloride responsive metabolic alkalosis is most common as it is seen in patients with vomiting, use of diuretics and post hypercapnic syndrome. It also can be seen in patients with chronic respiratory acidosis because of hypoventilation. In patients with decreased respirations (hypoventilation) there is an increase in the hypoxic state of the patient. Chronic pulmonary disease increases the risk of metabolic alkalosis due to hypercapnia and hypoxemia.

Chloride resistant hypochloremia is seen in patients with hyperadrenocorticism, primary hyperaldosteronism. The increase in mineralocorticoid activity creates sodium retention and excretion of the chloride in the urine. This keeps

---

Box 3.2 Causes of hypochloremia (Source: Data from Mazzaferro 2013)

Pseudohypochloremia

Hypoadrenocorticism
Third spacing
- Congestive heart failure

True

Disease process
- Chronic respiratory acidosis
- Hyperadrenocorticism
- Upper GI obstruction with vomiting

Drug administration
- Loop diuretics
  - furosemide
  - thiazide
  - sodium bicarbonate

---

an imbalance of the sodium:chloride ratio, which will result in a persistent metabolic alkalosis until the underlying cause is resolved.

Clinical signs

Clinical signs of hypochloremia are primarily due to the underlying disease process and depend on the acid-base status of the patient. Hyperexcitability of muscles, weakness, tetany, twitching, and muscle cramps may be seen. In patients with concurrent hypokalemia, cardiac dysrhythmias may be noted.

Treatment

In patients with chloride responsive hypochloremia, the chloride lost must be replaced with the use of intravenous fluids containing chloride. Additionally, the patient must be provided supplemental potassium and sodium. It is important to note that the hypochloremia will not resolve if hypokalemia is present: both must be addressed simultaneously. If volume expansion without sodium is required, administration of ammonium chloride, potassium chloride, calcium chloride, or magnesium chloride may be indicated. Treatment of the underlying disease is imperative for the patient's recovery. Oxygen therapy for patients with chronic pulmonary disease should be performed with caution.

It must be remembered that when correcting for potassium deficits in patients with metabolic alkalemia products which do not contain chloride, such as potassium phosphate (KPO_4), will not correct the chloride deficits. A chloride salt (NaCl or KCl) should be administered so that the kidney can reabsorb the chloride with the sodium to maintain electroneutrality. In many cases, 0.45 or 0.9% NaCl with KCl is an ideal combination. Administration of NaCl alone will cause diuresis with potassium excretion, which may ultimately worsen the patient's condition. In all cases the proper ratio of sodium to chloride (3:2) must be restored to correct this acid-base abnormality.

References

DiBartola, S. (2012). *Fluid, Electrolyte, and Acid-Base Disorders in Small Animal Practice*, 4th ed. Oxford: Elsevier.

Irani, D. (2008). *Cerebrospinal Fluid in Clinical Practice*. Oxford: Elsevier.

Feldman, C. & Nelson, R. (2004). *Canine and Feline Endocrinology and Reproduction*, 3rd ed. St Louis, MO: Saunders.

Mazzaferro, E. (2013). *Small Animal Fluid Therapy, Acid-Base and Electrolyte Disorders: A Color Handbook*. London: Manson Publishing.

CHAPTER 4

Disorders of Potassium

Dave Cowan, BA, CVT, VTS (ECC)

Potassium is the most abundant intracellular cation in the body with approximately 140 mEq/L (98%) residing within the cells, while only 3.5–5.5 mEq/L (~2%) are outside of the cells. There are many roles that potassium plays in the body, including muscle contraction, fluid balance, cell growth, resting cell potential, and nerve signal transmission, to name a few (Box 4.1). Potassium imbalance can be the result of many different factors including renal failure, improper acid-base status, and lack of intake.

Regulation of potassium

About 90% of the ingested potassium is absorbed in the small intestines. The potassium is then translocated from the extracellular fluid (ECF) to the intracellular fluid (ICF) by the function of insulin and catecholamines such as epinephrine or norepinephrine. Excretion of potassium takes place mainly via the function of the kidneys (90–95%), with the remainder being excreted through the colon (5–10%). In the kidneys, potassium is resorbed in the proximal convoluted tubule (PCT; ~60–70%), and thick ascending limb of the loop of Henle (LoH; ~20%). The remaining 10–15% of filtered potassium will reach the distal convoluted tubule (DCT). The DCT further controls the regulation of potassium by excreting or resorbing the potassium based on the body's overall potassium concentrations. Diuresis can cause increased potassium excretion, leading to hypokalemia, especially if the fluids being administered are potassium-deficient. Increased concentrations of potassium will stimulate aldosterone release from the adrenal glands, which will promote retention of sodium and excretion of potassium. When potassium concentrations are low, aldosterone release is not stimulated and more potassium can be resorbed in the DCT. Dietary

Acid-Base and Electrolyte Handbook for Veterinary Technicians, First Edition.
Edited by Angela Randels-Thorp and David Liss.
© 2017 John Wiley & Sons, Inc. Published 2017 by John Wiley & Sons, Inc.
Companion website: www.wiley.com/go/liss/electrolytes

Box 4.1 Roles of potassium

- Cell growth
- Maintenance of resting membrane potential
- Fluid balance
- Acid-base balance
- Electrolyte balance
- Muscle contraction
- Nerve signal transmission
- Glycogen and protein synthesis
- Blood pressure balance

---

potassium, after being absorbed through the gastrointestinal tract, is initially translocated from the ECF to the ICF. This movement is facilitated by insulin and catecholamines. Renal excretion will then normalize these levels over the following two days. If hyperkalemia is present, aldosterone will stimulate the colon to excrete potassium. The colon can also adapt by decreasing the secretion of potassium in the stool in cases of hypokalemia. The body's pH or acid-base status also plays a role in potassium excretion. Alkalosis will result in an excretion of potassium while retaining hydrogen ions. Acidosis will have the opposite effect, resorbing potassium while excreting hydrogen ions in the form of bicarbonate (HCO_3^-) (Aronson & Giebisch 2011).

Na+/K+-ATPase pump

The sodium-potassium adenosine triphosphatase pump (Na^+/K^+-ATPase) plays an important role in maintaining potassium balance in the body. Normal function of this process is vital for homeostasis. Hormones like insulin, epinephrine, norepinephrine, and thyroxine can stimulate the activity of the Na^+/K^+-ATPase pump. During this process, sodium and potassium are exchanged while ATP serves as the source of energy for the cell. The process involves the exchange of three sodium ions for two potassium ions from within the cell to outside the cell (Figure 4.1).

Three sodium ions will bind to the inside of the pump from within the cell while ATP is bound to the outside. The ATP then becomes hydrolyzed, forming ADP (adenosine diphosphate) and releasing energy for the cell as one of the phosphate ions breaks off and remains attached to the pump. The channel then changes shape, opening up to the extracellular space. The three sodium ions are released into the extracellular space, while two potassium ions bind to the inside of the pump. The remaining phosphate ion is then released from the pump, causing it to revert to its original shape where the potassium ions are released to the inside of the cell. ATP then binds to the pump restarting the process.

The Na^+/K^+-ATPase pump is essential for maintaining resting cell potential. While potassium is the most abundant intracellular cation, sodium is the most abundant extracellular cation (~150 mEq/L). The Na^+/K^+-ATPase pump helps

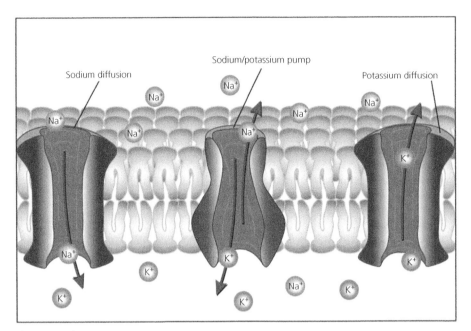

Figure 4.1 The Na$^+$/K$^+$-ATPase pump.

maintain this balance. Exchanging three positive ions for two positive ions leaves the cytoplasm of the cell with a relatively negative charge which is important for creating the cell's action potential. This negative charge is used in neurons and muscle cells for nerve function and muscle contraction. The pump is also important for maintaining cell volume by controlling the osmolality of the intracellular and extracellular spaces. In intracellular hyperosmolar states, fluid will shift into the cells, causing a decreased concentration of potassium within the cell, and potassium will flow back into the cell while sodium flows out. In extracellular hyperosmolar states, fluid shifts out of the cell to help reduce plasma osmolality. That shift of fluid results in an increased concentration of potassium within the cell that the Na$^+$/K$^+$-ATPase pump will correct by shifting potassium out into the extracellular space. If there is a decreased amount of potassium available within the cell, the cell becomes less excitable because less sodium will be able to flow in. If there is more potassium available within the cell, the resting cell potential will move closer to the threshold because more sodium can move into the cell making the cell more excitable. Once the threshold potential is exceeded, the cell cannot repolarize or depolarize. This scenario becomes life threatening especially when this happens in the myocardial cells.

Similar to the Na$^+$/K$^+$-ATPase pump, there is also a hydrogen-potassium adenosine triphosphatase pump (H$^+$/K$^+$-ATPase pump). ATP serves as the energy source for the cell, while hydrogen and potassium ions are exchanged in response to pH levels. Increased pH levels result in movement of potassium ions intracellularly, while hydrogen ions move to the extracellular space to reduce pH.

Conversely, decreased pH levels will shift potassium ions extracellularly, while hydrogen ions move intracellularly to increase pH (Gumz et al. 2010).

Hypokalemia

Causes of hypokalemia

When serum potassium concentration decreases below the normal range (3.5–5.5 mEq/L), the patient is in a state of hypokalemia. There are many causes for hypokalemia but most are attributed to either abnormal renal excretion or abnormal GI loss (Box 4.2). Anorexia will obviously cause a decreased intake of potassium and subsequently result in hypokalemia if allowed to persist over time. Increased GI loss (vomiting and/or diarrhea) will result in a decreased absorption of potassium as well as excessive elimination of potassium via the colon.

Given that the kidneys are the main source of potassium excretion, excessive urinary loss could be the cause of hypokalemia. Patients that are polyuric/polydipsic (PU/PD) can develop hypokalemia by drinking excessively and urinating excessively. The excessive water intake increases urinary production, which also means an increase in urinary excretion of potassium. In cases of urinary obstruction, potassium concentrations increase because it cannot be excreted. However, once the obstruction is cleared and the animal is administered intravenous fluids, the diuresis can bring potassium concentrations back down to below normal ranges, called post-obstructive hypokalemia. Patients that are given intravenous fluids for any reason can develop hypokalemia if the fluids do not contain appropriate concentrations of potassium.

Insulin activates the Na^+/K^+-ATPase pump, which will drive potassium into the cells and can cause an abnormally low serum concentration. Refeeding syndrome is a condition where an animal that has not eaten for a prolonged period (7–10 days) is then re-introduced to food. As a result of this refeeding, electrolyte disturbances will occur. During the starvation/malnourishment period,

---

Box 4.2 Causes of hypokalemia

- Decreased intake
- Increased intracellular translocation
- Increased gastrointestinal loss
- Increased urinary loss
- Hypothyroidism
- Hypothermia
- Metabolic alkalosis
- Drug administration
- Hyperadrenocorticism (Cushing's disease)
- Rattlesnake envenomation

insulin concentrations will decrease while glucagon increases. The body tries to preserve muscle and protein breakdown by converting to ketone production as a result of fat metabolism, as a replacement energy source. Cells become depleted of magnesium, phosphates, and potassium due to a lack of intake, while plasma concentrations can remain normal. Once feeding is reintroduced, insulin is released in response to the increase of glucose. Insulin then drives magnesium, phosphorus, glucose, and potassium back into the depleted cells, causing plasma concentrations to drop dangerously low.

The administration of certain drugs can also cause potassium concentrations to drop. Loop diuretics, which act on the ascending LoH, such as furosemide or thiazide diuretics such as hydrochlorothiazide, can promote potassium excretion leading to hypokalemia. Albuterol, which is a bronchodilator that works by beta-adrenergic agonism, will activate the Na^+/K^+-ATPase pump, driving potassium intracellularly. Nephrotoxic drugs such as the antifungal medication amphotericin B can cause hypokalemia by slowing the glomerular filtration rate (GFR) of the kidney. The slower GFR results in less potassium delivery to the DCT where excretion or resorption takes place.

Patients experiencing metabolic alkalosis can become hypokalemic. The body is constantly trying to achieve and maintain homeostasis. In states of alkalosis, where pH is increased, hydrogen ions shift out of the intracellular space into the extracellular space in exchange for potassium ions in an effort to reduce plasma pH. There is an increased concentration of HCO_3^- (bicarbonate) during states of metabolic alkalosis. The kidneys will excrete the excess bicarbonate along with potassium ions (in addition to the lungs decreasing excretion of carbon dioxide) to help lower pH levels.

Hyperadrenocorticism (Cushing's disease) will cause an excess of adrenocorticotropic hormone (ACTH) which makes the adrenal glands produce too much cortisol and corticosteroids. Cortisol will stimulate gluconeogenesis, which will raise the glucose level, which in turn will stimulate more insulin release. As we discussed earlier, insulin helps drive glucose and potassium into the cells. An increase in aldosterone can also cause hypokalemia. One of the roles of aldosterone is to promote sodium retention and potassium excretion. In patients with an excess of aldosterone there will be decreased potassium and increased sodium plasma concentrations. This scenario will cause a fluid shift from the intracellular space to the extracellular space to reduce sodium concentration, leading to hypertension and hypokalemia.

Clinical signs

Hypokalemic patients can develop a variety of clinical complications, the most obvious being skeletal muscle weakness. The feline patient with low potassium concentrations will often present with ventroflexion of the neck. Potassium concentrations less than 3.0 mEq/L will contribute to the overall muscle weakness and ventroflexion. A plantigrade stance, where the patient will stand with its hocks resting on the ground, may also be noted. Potassium deficiency causes a disturbance at the neuromuscular junction due to impaired electrical conduction at the cell membrane level. Skeletal muscle weakness can lead to a decreased muscle mass and weight loss. Patients with serum potassium concentrations of less than 2.0 mEq/L can develop rhabdomyolysis. Rhabdomyolysis is a condition where muscle tissue breaks down and the intracellular contents such as the protein myoglobin and the enzyme creatine kinase are released into the bloodstream. The breakdown of myoglobin can cause acute renal failure due to the toxic effects it has on the kidneys.

Cardiac arrhythmias can occur when potassium concentrations are below 2.5 mEq/L. Decreased concentrations of potassium will cause a prolonged repolarization of the ventricular Purkinje fibers. With lower potassium concentrations, the cells become less excitable because there is less potassium available to flow into the cells. There can be many ECG abnormalities, including increased P wave amplitude, depressed ST elevation, decreased or inverted T wave, appearance of a U wave, sinus bradycardia, heart block, and prolonged PR interval, QT interval, and QRS complexes. If hypokalemia is allowed to continue or progress, ventricular arrhythmias may develop, potentially leading to ventricular fibrillation. Torsades de pointes (French for "twisting of spikes" or "twisting of points") is a ventricular tachycardia that can arise from hypokalemia. The QRS complexes will vary in duration and amplitude, giving the appearance of a twisted ribbon on the ECG strip. This variation in QRS complexes is a result of prolonged QT intervals. The QT interval represents the time between ventricular depolarization and ventricular repolarization, which will be prolonged during states of hypokalemia.

Metabolic alkalosis can be a complication of hypokalemia as well as a cause of hypokalemia. Decreased potassium concentrations will activate the H^+/K^+-ATPase pumps, pushing potassium extracellularly while shifting hydrogen intracellularly. The resulting increase in intracellular hydrogen ions means that more hydrogen ions are available for excretion in the renal tubules. This will promote renal tubular bicarbonate resorption in an effort to raise pH levels leading to a metabolic alkalosis.

Treatment of hypokalemia

The treatment of hypokalemia involves replacing the potassium deficits while also making an effort to treat the underlying cause or causes. Potassium can be supplemented either enterally or parenterally. Potassium gluconate can be fed orally or through a feeding tube at the dose of 2 mEq/4.5 kg twice daily. Potassium gluconate is available in capsule, tablet, powder, and paste form. Foods that are rich in potassium can also be fed to help replenish potassium deficiencies. Sweet potatoes and bananas contain over 400 mg of potassium which roughly calculates to 10 mEq. While feeding potassium-rich foods can help, it is not an accurate means of potassium supplementation. Patients that cannot be supplemented enterally will require parenteral supplementation with potassium chloride added to intravenous fluids

Table 4.1 Recommended potassium supplementation

Serum potassium level (mEq/L)	Potassium chloride added to crystalloid fluid (mEq)
<2	80
2.0–2.5	60
2.5–3.0	40
3.0–3.5	30
3.5–4.0	20

(Table 4.1). It is important to ensure that potassium is replaced at a rate not to exceed 0.5 mEq/kg/hr for patients with mild to moderate hypokalemia as there is a risk of causing cardiac conduction changes as well as making the patient hyperkalemic with over supplementation (Plumb 2008). Patients with more profound hypokalemia (<2.0 mEq/L) can be supplemented at a higher rate (up to 1.0 mEq/kg/hr) but should be carefully monitored for signs of hyperkalemia using re-evaluation of potassium concentrations and continuous ECG monitoring.

Hyperkalemia

Causes

When serum potassium concentration rises above the normal range (3.5–5.5 mEq/L), the patient is in a state of hyperkalemia. The kidneys are very efficient at maintaining potassium balance, so it is rare to have a patient with hyperkalemia that has normal kidney function. Patients with oliguric renal failure or patients with a urinary obstruction will have increased potassium concentrations because the kidneys are not able to excrete it normally.

Adrenal insufficiency can be responsible for a patient to present with increased serum potassium concentrations. Hypoadrenocorticism, or Addison's disease, occurs when the adrenal glands do not produce sufficient amounts of glucocorticoids or mineralocorticoids either from damaged adrenal glands or from a lack of adrenocorticotrophic hormone (ACTH) production from the pituitary gland. Patients with Addison's disease will often present with hypercalcemia, hypoglycemia, hyponatremia, and hyperkalemia. The mineralocorticoid aldosterone is responsible for maintaining electrolyte and fluid balance. This is done by activation of the Na^+/K^+-ATPase pump where sodium and water are resorbed while potassium is excreted in the kidneys. Without the presence of aldosterone, potassium will be resorbed, and sodium and water will be excreted, leading to dehydration, hyponatremia, and hyperkalemia.

Diabetic patients that are also experiencing ketoacidosis (DKA) may initially present with increased potassium concentrations. Dehydration, decreased insulin, and acidemia are all factors contributing to this hyperkalemic state. DKA patients commonly present with vomiting, leading to dehydration, which will cause an increased potassium concentration. A lack of insulin will contribute additionally to increased potassium concentrations, owing to the lack of Na^+/K^+-ATPase pump activation. Acidemic states will result in hyperkalemia as the increased hydrogen ion concentrations will activate the H^+/K^+-ATPase pumps, forcing potassium extracellularly. After rehydration and treatment of the acidosis, however, these patients will actually become hypokalemic. Shifting of potassium due to the reasons outlined above result in a total body deficit intracellularly. Diuresis will further reduce potassium concentrations by dilution, insulin administration will drive potassium back into the cells by activation of the Na^+/K^+-ATPase pumps, and correction of the acidemia can reveal an overall severe hypokalemia.

Iatrogenic over supplementation of potassium can also be a cause of hyperkalemia. Over supplementation due to excessive intake is rare. Potassium is quickly redistributed into the cells via insulin until the kidneys are able to excrete the excess over time, so excessive intake is an unlikely cause of over supplementation. Patients being supplemented with intravenous fluids containing potassium additives such as potassium chloride or potassium phosphate can have elevated potassium concentrations if being supplemented at high rates for long duration or if the rate of potassium administration exceeds the recommended 0.5–1.0 mEq/kg/hr dose.

Drug administration can contribute to increased potassium concentrations. Spironolactone is a potassium-sparing diuretic given to help promote diuresis, but also to prevent excessive potassium excretion. Increased potassium resorption due to potassium-sparing agents can cause elevated concentrations. Digoxin can cause increased potassium concentrations because it will compete with the potassium ions for the same spot in the Na^+/K^+-ATPase pump. Beta-blockers (propranolol, atenolol, etc.) are drugs used to decrease heart rate and cause vasodilation by antagonizing the beta-receptors. Beta-receptor agonism helps to promote the activity of the Na^+/K^+-ATPase pump. Antagonizing these beta-receptors will decrease the exchange of potassium ions for sodium ions, leading to an increased concentration of potassium in the ECF. Angiotensin-converting enzyme (ACE) inhibitors (such as enalapril) block the conversion of angiotensin I to angiotensin II. One of the major roles of angiotensin II is to stimulate the adrenal glands to produce aldosterone. When this process is inhibited, there will be a decreased level of aldosterone production. Decreased aldosterone levels will lead to an increased potassium resorption in the kidneys. Non-steroidal anti-inflammatory drugs (NSAIDs; ibuprofen, carprofen, etc.), or any drug that can be nephrotoxic, will obviously have an impact on renal excretion of potassium.

Clinical signs

Complications from hyperkalemia can be seen when plasma potassium concentrations rise above 7.5–8.0 mEq/L. As discussed before, hypokalemia can cause a metabolic alkalosis. The inverse is also true. Hyperkalemia can result in a metabolic

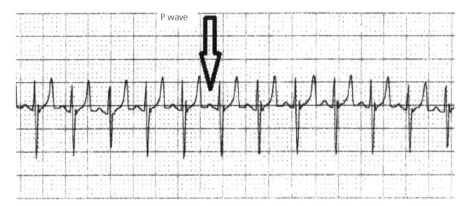

Figure 4.2 ECG changes due to hyperkalemia, tall, spiked T-waves.

acidosis. The increased potassium concentration activates the H^+/K^+-ATPase pump shifting potassium ions intracellularly, while hydrogen ions shift extracellularly in an effort to increase plasma pH. Hyperkalemic patients will often present with muscular weakness, abdominal pain, diarrhea, and cardiac abnormalities.

Cardiac arrhythmias will occur with hyperkalemia, owing to the increased extracellular potassium causing changes in the resting membrane potential of the myocardial cells (Parham et al., 2006). The potassium-sodium concentration gradient between the intracellular and extracellular space is important for maintaining normal myocardial cell function. Changes can be seen on an electrocardiogram (Figure 4.2), the first being tall, peaked T waves, which represent ventricular repolarization. With higher potassium concentrations, the cell membranes become more excitable and have a much shorter repolarization period, which is represented by the tall, peaked T waves. With higher potassium levels, the myocardial cells of the atria are unable to depolarize, resulting in the progressive flattening of the P waves to the point where they disappear. When P waves disappear (Figure 4.3), there is no atrial contraction and the heart relies on the AV node or Purkinje's fibers to be the pacemaker. This will cause a prolonged QRS complex and bradycardia. Progression of these abnormalities can eventually lead to ventricular fibrillation and cardiac arrest.

Pseudohyperkalemia

Serum potassium concentrations can be falsely elevated, owing to leakage from increased numbers of potassium-containing cells. Patients with severe leukocytosis or thrombocytosis can exhibit elevated levels of serum potassium. Hemolysis, which can occur from improper blood-drawing technique or sample handling, can cause pseudohyperkalemia, owing to the destruction of blood cells which will release the intracellular potassium into the serum. Acute tumor lysis syndrome also causes the destruction of potassium-containing cancer cells, which will elevate serum potassium concentrations. Any destruction of

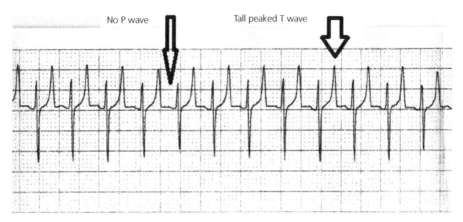

No P wave   Tall peaked T wave

Figure 4.3 ECG changes related to increasing hyperkalemia.

potassium-containing cells has the potential to elevate serum potassium concentration levels and give the appearance of hyperkalemia.

Treatment of hyperkalemia

As with all electrolyte and laboratory abnormalities, the main goal of treatment is not only to correct the abnormalities but also to treat the underlying cause of the issue. Hyperkalemia is not a disease in and of itself, but more a result of some condition or disease process. Intravenous fluids may be an adequate treatment if the potassium concentration is moderately elevated (6.0–8.0 mEq/L). Simple diuresis may be enough to bring potassium concentrations down into the normal range. Second, adding dextrose with or without insulin will drive the potassium back into the cells. Potassium will follow glucose into the cells through the function of insulin and its effect on the Na$^+$/K$^+$-ATPase pump. Dextrose is given at a dose of 0.5–1 gm/kg and can be followed with regular insulin at a dose of 0.5–1.1 U/kg. Diuretics such as furosemide can be given to help promote diuresis, provided that the patient has normal kidney function (Norkus 2012).

Patients with severely increased potassium concentrations (>8.0 mEq/L) that have cardiac arrhythmias will require calcium gluconate to protect the myocardial cells (Parham et al. 2006). Calcium gluconate will antagonize the effects of the increased potassium concentration, allowing the myocardial cells to have normal excitability. Decreasing the difference between the resting potential and threshold potential of the myocardial cells will stabilize the membranes and allow for more normal excitability. Administration of calcium gluconate will restore some normal myocardial function, most notably the reappearance of P waves (Figure 4.3). When cardiac dysrhythmias of hyperkalemic origin are found, calcium gluconate should be given at 50–100 mg/kg IV over 10–20 minutes (Plumb 2008). It should be noted that calcium gluconate does *not* have any effect on the potassium concentration, but rather protects the myocardium. The effects of calcium gluconate administration have a quick onset, but only a short period of duration (10–15 minutes). Monitoring of the patient's ECG should be done to evaluate efficacy of calcium gluconate administration.

In cases of severe hyperkalemia that are also severely acidotic (pH < 7.1), sodium bicarbonate can be administered [0.3 × BW(kg) × base excess]. Sodium bicarbonate will increase the pH level, which will help push potassium back into the cells in exchange for hydrogen ions by activation of the H^+/K^+-ATPase pump. Administration of sodium bicarbonate can have adverse effects and should be administered with caution. It is recommended to give half the calculated dose as a constant rate infusion over 4–6 hr, or possibly as bolus over 30–60 minutes if the patient is in a life-threatening state. Acid-base status should be re-evaluated after administration. The administration of the second half of the dose should be considered if the patient is persistently acidemic and hyperkalemic. Care should be taken whenever administering sodium bicarbonate. If the patient has an altered level of consciousness and is unable to adjust their ventilation rate, CO_2 given off as a byproduct will build up in the bloodstream to elevated levels and the patient may become hypercapneic. The blood–brain barrier is very sensitive to CO_2 and cerebral acidosis may result. This can cause coma or even death in a critically ill patient. Over administration of sodium bicarbonate will potentially cause metabolic alkalosis, which can lead to many additional complications. Increased plasma pH can decrease the ability of hemoglobin to unload its oxygen load into the cells. Calcium levels can be decreased, owing to calcium's affinity to bind to albumin when pH levels are elevated. Decreased calcium levels can lead to tetany and cardiac arrhythmias. When pH levels are elevated, the body will compensate by trying to retain more carbon dioxide. In order to retain more carbon dioxide, the respiratory drive can be decreased, leading to hypoventilation, and may require mechanical ventilation. The hypernatremia that can result from the addition of sodium will create a hyperosmolarity in the plasma, causing a fluid shift from the intracellular space to the extracellular space putting the patient at risk for fluid overload as well as cellular dehydration.

Acid-/Base disturbances and potassium

When evaluating a patient's acid-base status, pH, carbon dioxide, and bicarbonate are commonly considered. Approaches to acid-base determination are discussed in other chapters in this text. Potassium concentrations can also provide a look into the acid-base status of the patient. Acid-base disturbances involving potassium disorders are generally related to the metabolic forms. Respiratory forms of acid-base disturbances rely on the lungs for the regulation of carbon dioxide levels. Metabolic forms of acid-base disturbances rely on renal regulation of bicarbonate and potassium. When there is an alkalemia or acidemia, the body corrects this by shifting hydrogen ions from the intracellular and extracellular spaces in exchange for potassium ions by activation of the H^+/K^+-ATPase pump.

In metabolic alkalosis, pH is elevated; there is a decreased amount of extracellular hydrogen ions and an increased bicarbonate concentration. The kidneys will excrete the excess bicarbonate, along with potassium ions. Hydrogen ions will shift from the intracellular space into the extracellular space by activation of the H^+/K^+-ATPase pump to decrease pH. As a result of this process, patients with metabolic alkalosis will generally have a concurrent hypokalemia.

Metabolic acidosis is the most common acid-base disturbance and is caused by a loss of bicarbonate resulting in a decreased pH level. During metabolic acidosis, the higher hydrogen ion concentrations will activate the H^+/K^+-ATPase pump, pushing hydrogen ions intracellularly, while potassium ions are pushed extracellularly. As a result of this process, patients with metabolic acidosis will have increased potassium concentrations.

Use of the anion gap equation to determine the cause of metabolic acidosis involves the use of potassium concentrations. Plasma always maintains an electroneutrality, meaning that, overall, there is neither a positive nor a negative charge. We know that the amount of cations (positively charged ions) and the anions (negatively charged ions) will be equal. Calculating the difference between measurable cations (sodium and potassium) and measureable anions (bicarbonate and chloride) will give us an indication of the cause of the metabolic acidosis. An elevated anion gap (>15 mmol/L) indicates there is an excessive amount of unmeasured acids in the plasma. Elevated anion gaps are commonly seen in lactic acidosis and diabetic ketoacidosis and can also be seen with ethylene glycol intoxication. Normal anion gaps will indicate that the cause of the acidosis is primarily from a loss of bicarbonate.

Summary

In summary, potassium disorders are most commonly associated with renal insufficiency, as the kidneys are primarily responsible for the regulation of potassium balance. Severe complications can arise from improper regulation of potassium, most commonly from an increase or decrease in excretion. There is a very narrow range of what is considered the normal plasma potassium concentration (3.5–5.5 mEq/L). The body is very efficient at keeping potassium concentrations within that normal range. However, when the body cannot control this balance, the veterinary team needs to intervene and help bring potassium concentrations back into the normal range. Supplementation of potassium can lead to hyperkalemia and all of its complications if given too rapidly. Efforts to reduce potassium concentrations can potentially bring potassium concentrations below the normal range as a result of dilution when using diuresis. Methods which promote cellular uptake of potassium can also bring serum concentrations below the normal range as well. Our interventions can have adverse effects if they are not done correctly (Scalf 2014).

References

Aronson, P. & Giebisch, G. (2011). Effects of pH on potassium: New explanations for old observations. *Journal of the American Society of Nephrology* **22**(11): 1981–9.

Gumz, M. et al. (2010). The renal H^+-K^+-ATPases: Physiology, regulation, and structure. *American Journal of Physiology Renal Physiology* **298**(1): F12–F21.

Norkus, C. (ed.) (2012). *Veterinary Technician's Manual for Small Animal Emergency and Critical Care*. Ames, IA: Wiley-Blackwell.

Parham, W. et al. (2006). Hyperkalemia revisited. *Texas Heart Institute Journal* **33**(1): 40–47.

Plumb, D. (2008). *Plumb's Veterinary Drug Handbook*, 6th ed. Ames, IA: Blackwell Publishing.

Scalf, R. (ed.) (2014). *Study Guide to the AVECCT Examination*, 2nd ed. San Antonio, TX: VECCS Publishing.

Further reading

DiBartola, S. (2011). *Fluid, Electrolyte, and Acid-Base Disorders in Small Animal Practice*, 4th ed. St Louis, MO: Elsevier Saunders.

Ettinger, S. & Feldman, E. (eds), (2010). *Textbook of Veterinary Internal Medicine*, 7th ed. St Louis MO: Elsevier Saunders.

Silverstein, D. & Hopper, K. (eds) (2009). *Small Animal Critical Care Medicine*. St Louis, MO: Elsevier Saunders.

CHAPTER 5

Disorders of Magnesium

Louise O'Dwyer, MBA, BSc (Hons), VTS (Anaesthesia & ECC),
DipAVN (Medical & Surgical), RVN

Disorders of magnesium

Magnesium (Mg$^+$) is the second most abundant intracellular cation, exceeded only by potassium, and the fourth most abundant total cation (Martin et al. 1993). Sixty percent of the total body magnesium content is present in bone, incorporated in the crystal mineral lattice or in the surface limited exchangeable pool. Twenty percent is located in skeletal muscle, while the remainder exists in other tissues, primarily the heart and liver (Berkelhammer & Bear 1985). Only about 1% is located extracellularly in the serum and interstitial body fluid. Extra-cellular magnesium is present in three forms: an ionized form that is biologically active (55%), a protein-bound form (20–30%), and an anion-complex form (15–25%). The ionized fraction is believed to be the physiologically active component. Magnesium is only 20–30% bound to protein, being less affected by changes in albumin concentration than calcium. Magnesium is regulated in the gastrointestinal tract and kidneys under the influence of parathyroid hormone and 1,25-dihydroxycholecalciferol. Increased morbidity and mortality can occur in critically ill patients with altered serum magnesium concentrations.

Magnesium has a vital role in numerous metabolic functions, most importantly those involved in the production and use of adenosine triphosphate (ATP). It is a co-enzyme for sodium-potassium ATPase, calcium ATPase, and proton pumps (Whang & Ryder 1990). Magnesium is the naturally occurring antagonist to calcium and their absorption is interdependent (Jenkinson 1957). Magnesium functions to maintain the sodium-potassium gradient across all membranes. It also regulates intracellular calcium levels by its calcium channel-blocking effects. Interference with these gradients may result in changes in the resting membrane potential and disturbances in depolarization. This highlights magnesium's pivotal role in both muscle contraction and cardiac conduction (Martin et al. 1993).

Acid-Base and Electrolyte Handbook for Veterinary Technicians, First Edition.
Edited by Angela Randels-Thorp and David Liss.
© 2017 John Wiley & Sons, Inc. Published 2017 by John Wiley & Sons, Inc.
Companion website: www.wiley.com/go/liss/electrolytes

Magnesium also participates in the regulation of vascular smooth muscle tone, cellular second messenger systems, and signal transduction. In addition, recent data suggest magnesium exerts an important influence on lymphocyte activation and cytokine production.

Magnesium homeostasis is achieved through intestinal absorption and renal excretion. The absorption of magnesium occurs primarily in the ileum, but the jejunum and colon also contribute substantially to net absorption (Bateman 2008). At this time several key mechanism are understood regarding the absorption of magnesium from the ileum, with it being determined that two pathways for absorption exist: an unsaturable passive paracellular route and a saturable active transcellular route (Bateman 2012). The paracellular movement of magnesium is via the tight junctions between epithelial cells, with the driving forces for this movement being the transepithelial magnesium concentration gradient formed by salt and water absorption, and the permeability of the tight junctions to magnesium (Bateman 2012).

The kidney appears to be the main regulator of serum magnesium concentration, balance, and total body magnesium content. This is achieved by both glomerular filtration and tubular reabsorption (Sachter 1992). Various areas of the nephron play an important role in magnesium homeostasis. Around 80% of total serum magnesium is filtered by the glomerulus and enters the proximal tubule (DiBartola 2012). Of the filtered magnesium: 10–15% is reabsorbed within the proximal tubule, 60–70% is reabsorbed in the cortical thick ascending limb of the loop of Henle, and 10–15% is reabsorbed in the distal convoluted tubule (DCT). The final concentration of magnesium in the urine is determined at the DCT, which is under both hormonal and non-hormonal control (Bateman 2008). Renal magnesium excretion will increase in proportion to the magnesium load presented to the kidney; conversely, the kidney conserves magnesium in response to a deficiency (Friday & Reinhart 1990).

As a predominantly intracellular cation, the study of magnesium balance has been difficult due to the limited correlation between the readily measurable, but relatively small, circulating fraction of serum magnesium. Less than 1% of the total body magnesium is present in the serum, and these serum concentrations may not accurately reflect total body stores of magnesium, with serum magnesium levels appearing normal despite total body depletion.

Magnesium concentrations are very tightly controlled within the body. Both total (tMg) and ionized (iMg) magnesium concentrations can be measured. Total magnesium levels are fairly stable and can be measured from either a serum or heparinized whole blood sample. Table 5.1 lists the normal ranges for tMg and iMg. Total magnesium levels can be measured using the IDEXX VetTest analyzer. Similar to calcium, iMg levels can be measured using ion-selective electrodes. The iMg level will be lower than the tMg level. Ionized magnesium can be measured on certain NOVA analyzers. Similarly to measuring potassium, a low magnesium concentration suggests that total body stores are

Table 5.1 Normal magnesium levels in dogs and cats (Source: Adapted from Firth 2010)

	mmol/l	mg/dl	mEq/l
tMg (dog)	0.7–1.0	1.6–2.5	1.4–2.0
iMg (dog)	0.43–0.6	—	—
tMg (cat)	0.8–1.0	1.9–2.6	1.6–2.0
iMg (cat)	0.43–0.7	—	—

depleted. Conversely, intracellular magnesium levels may be low even though serum magnesium is normal. Ionized magnesium levels can be negatively affected by the administration of many anions that are commonly administered or increased in critically ill patients, such as heparin, citrate, lactate, bicarbonate, phosphate, acetate and sulfate (Wingfield 2002).

The interpretation of magnesium levels can sometimes be difficult and confusing, as magnesium concentrations can be reported in different units. A magnesium level of 1 mmol/L equates to 2.43 mg/dL. To convert mmol/L to mg/dL, multiply by 2.43. To convert mg/dL to mmol/L, multiply by 0.411. Magnesium levels are sometimes reported in mEq/L. Since magnesium is a divalent cation, 1 mmol/L is 2 mEq/L (Firth 2010).

The relevance of magnesium in the majority of veterinary practice may be severely underestimated. In a 1994 study of 48 dogs by Martin et al. (1993), the incidence of hypomagnesemia (tMg <1.89 mg/dL) was 54% highlighting the need to consider hypomagnesemia in the critical patient population.

Hypomagnesemia

Hypomagnesemia encountered more commonly than hypermagnesemia, and has been reported to occur in approximately 54% of critically ill veterinary patients, establishing hypomagnesemia as one of the most clinically significant electrolyte disorders in critically ill patients (Martin et al. 1994). There are numerous causes of hypomagnesemia, but they are generally divided into: decreased intake, increased losses, and alteration in distribution. Decreased dietary intake of magnesium, if sustained for several weeks, can lead to significant magnesium depletion. In addition, catabolic illness and prolonged intravenous fluid therapy or parenteral nutrition without magnesium supplementation can contribute to magnesium depletion (Firth 2010).

Increased magnesium losses may occur through the gastrointestinal tract or via the kidneys. Increased gastrointestinal losses of magnesium may result from inflammatory bowel disease, malabsorptive syndromes, cholestatic liver disease, or other diseases that cause prolonged diarrhea (Martin & Allen-Durrance 2015).

The primary pathway of magnesium excretion is the kidney, and as such it often serves as a focal point for the development of hypomagnesemia as a result of urinary loss of magnesium. Acute renal dysfunction as a consequence of glomerulonephritis, or the non-oliguric phase of acute tubular necrosis, is often associated with a rise in the fractional excretion of magnesium. A number of endocrinopathies are also associated with an increase in the fractional excretion of magnesium, including diabetic ketoacidosis and hyperthyroidism. Disease states, or therapeutic modalities, may cause the redistribution of circulating magnesium by producing extracellular to intracellular shifts, chelation, or sequestration; examples include blood transfusion or disease states, such as pancreatitis, refeeding syndrome, and sepsis (Cortés & Moses 2007).

Numerous drugs administered to emergency and critically ill patients may also increase renal magnesium loss. Most of the commonly administered diuretic agents (furosemide, thiazides, mannitol) and cardiac glycosides induce hypomagnesemia by increasing urinary magnesium excretion. Other drugs—such as aminoglycosides, amphotericin B, and cisplatin—predispose to renal tubular injury and excessive magnesium loss (Table 5.2).

Table 5.2 Causes of magnesium deficit (Source: Based on data from Martin & Allen-Durrance 2015)

Gastrointestinal	Renal	Miscellaneous
Decreased intake	Diabetes mellitus/diabetic ketoacidosis	Excessive loss via: • Sweating • Lactation
Chronic diarrhea	Diuretics (except potassium sparing agents)	Redistribution Acute myocardial infarction Acute pancreatitis Insulin Catecholamine release
Malabsorption Short bowel syndrome	Osmotic agents (including hyperglycemia) Intrinsic renal causes Post-obstructive Polyuric acute failure Hyperaldosteronism Hyperthyroidism	Idiopathic
Familial or inherited	Concurrent electrolyte disorders Hypokalemia Hypercalcemia/hyperparathyroidism Hypophosphatemia Drugs • Gentamycin • Carbenicillin • Ticarcillin • Cyclosporine • Cisplatin Familial or inherited	

Clinical signs

The clinical signs associated with magnesium depletion are often related to its effects on the cell membrane, which result in changes in the resting membrane potential, signal transduction, and smooth muscle tone. Magnesium acts as a regulator of other ions, primarily calcium and potassium, and it this role of regulator that results in the effects of magnesium on the myocardium. Due to these effects, one of the most dramatic clinical signs associated with hypomagnesemia is cardiac arrhythmia. Such arrhythmias include atrial fibrillation, supraventricular tachycardia, ventricular tachycardia, and ventricular fibrillation. Hypomagnesemia also predisposes patients to digitalis-induced arrhythmias. This is because it not only enhances digitalis uptake by the myocardium but also inhibits the myocardial sodium-potassium ATPase pump, as does digitalis. Before arrhythmia development is observed, ECG changes may be seen. These include prolongation of the PR interval, widening of the QRS complex, depression of the ST segment, and peaking of the T wave.

Magnesium deficiency can result in a variety of non-specific neuromuscular signs, which may be further compounded by concurrent hypocalcemia and hypokalemia. Clinical manifestations of magnesium deficiency include skeletal muscle weakness, muscle fasciculation, seizures, and ataxia. Esophageal or respiratory muscle weakness can result in dysphagia or dyspnea, respectively.

Metabolic complications of hypomagnesemia include concurrent hypokalemia, hyponatremia, hypocalcemia, hypophosphatemia. Concurrent hypokalemia that is refractory to aggressive potassium supplementation may be due to a magnesium deficiency.

Treatment

The amount and route of magnesium replacement will be very much dependent on the degree of hypomagnesemia, from blood sampling, but also on the patient's clinical condition. If only mild hypomagnesemia is present, this may resolve with treatment of the underlying disorder and modification of intravenous fluid therapy.

In patients that are receiving long-term diuretic and digoxin, oral magnesium supplementation may be considered. Supplementation should be considered in any patient if serum magnesium levels are lower than 1.5 mg/dL (normal range for dogs is 1.89–2.51 mg/dL) and at any level if clinical signs (cardiac arrhythmias, muscle tremors, refractory hypokalemia) are present. Renal function and cardiac conduction should always be assessed prior to magnesium administration, and due to its mainly hepatic excretion, then in azotemic patients, supplementation should be reduced by 50%, and serum levels monitored frequently to prevent the development of hypermagnesemia. Magnesium also prolongs conduction through the AV node. Therefore, any patient with cardiac conduction disturbances should have judicious supplementation of magnesium and continuous ECG monitoring (Martin 2003).

Hypomagnesemia is generally treated via the infusion of magnesium sulfate ($MgSO_4$) or magnesium chloride ($MgCl_2$). Both magnesium sulfate and magnesium chloride are available in different concentrations (12.5–50% solutions) and due to the hyperosmolar nature of these solutions, it is recommended that they are diluted to a concentration less than 20% via dilution in either 0.9% NaCl or 5% dextrose in water (Bateman 2012). It should also be noted that calcium-, bicarbonate-, and lactate-containing solutions are incompatible with magnesium salt solutions (Humphrey et al. 2015).

The dose rate for magnesium supplementation varies between available texts, but the most current recommendation of magnesium sulfate in dogs and cats is 0.1–0.15 mmol/kg (0.2–0.3 mEq/kg) IV at a rate of 0.06 mmol/kg/min (0.12 mEq/kg/min) (Humphrey et al. 2015). This dose is recommended for treating acute, life-threatening problems associated with magnesium deficiency (e.g. Torsades de pointes and other cardiac arrhythmias). These dose rates are based on 1999 study by Nakayama et al.

A constant rate infusion (0.1–0.5 mmol/kg/day [0.2–1 mEq/kg/day]) may be required to treat magnesium-deficient animals that have ongoing magnesium loss or chronic magnesium deficiency (Humphrey et al. 2015).

During magnesium administration, patients should be carefully monitored for signs of magnesium toxicity, which can include vomiting, diarrhea, hypotension, weakness, and respiratory depression. Continuous ECG and blood pressure monitoring should be performed throughout administration because, as previously mentioned, hypotension can be seen, along with ECG abnormalities, which can include bradycardia, QT interval prolongation, PR interval prolongation, and QRS complex widening (Humphrey et al. 2015), atrioventricular and bundle-branch blocks (Martin 2003). These adverse effects, however, tend to be associated with intravenous boluses rather than continuous rate infusions.

Oral supplementation of magnesium can be accomplished with a variety of magnesium (chloride, gluconate, oxide, and hydroxide) salts. The recommended dose is 1–2 mEq/kg/day (Firth 2010). Diarrhea may be seen with oral supplementation since magnesium salts are cathartic.

In addition to monitoring plasma magnesium concentrations, plasma potassium, sodium, calcium, and chloride should also be monitored. The relationships between hypomagnesemia and other electrolyte disorders have been well documented and hypomagnesemia should be considered in cases of refractory hypokalemia and hypocalcemia.

Magnesium is used regularly in human medicine as an adjunct to therapy for a number of conditions including brain injury, spinal injury, pain, sepsis, and systemic inflammatory response syndrome, hypercoagulable states, eclampsia, tetanus, and ischemia (Humphrey et al. 2015). In these conditions magnesium is administered for its beneficial actions in specific cells. The author has successfully used magnesium sulfate in the treatment of autonomic dysfunction in a dog with severe generalized tetanus (Figure 5.1).

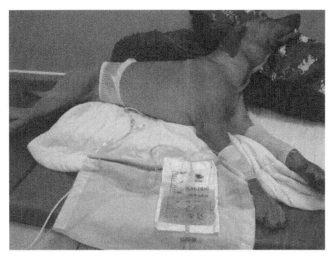

Figure 5.1 Patient with tetanus receiving a constant rate infusion of intravenous magnesium.

Hypermagnesemia

Hypermagnesemia is observed far less frequently compared to hypomagnesemia, and since it is readily excreted in the urine, provided patients have normal renal function it is rarely observed within veterinary practice. Hypermagnesemia, unsurprisingly, is seen in patients with renal failure or following overdose of magnesium sulfate or, less commonly, magnesium chloride. Overdose is more common again in patients with impaired renal function, where magnesium excretion is reduced.

Several endocrinopathies may be associated with hypermagnesemia. These diseases include hypoadrenocorticism, hyperparathyroidism, and hypothyroidism. In comparison with renal failure, these diseases cause hypermagnesemia less frequently and to a milder degree. The mechanisms that lead to hypermagnesemia are not well understood in these endocrine disorders (Martin 2003).

Clinical signs

The clinical signs associated with hypermagnesemia are fairly non-specific and can include lethargy, depression, and weakness. Other clinical signs as associated with the action of the ion on both the nervous and cardiovascular systems. Hypotension related to a loss of vascular resistance can occur because of the effect of magnesium on calcium channels. If hypermagnesemia is severe enough, respiratory depression can develop due to the neuromuscular-blocking effects of magnesium. The mechanism for this effect is high serum magnesium concentrations blocking the calcium-dependent release of acetylcholine at the presynaptic neuromuscular junction (Cortés & Moses 2007).

Hypermagnesemia can, of course, occur as a result of iatrogenic overdose. One of the first clinical signs associated with magnesium toxicity is hyporeflexia, which can progress, if undetected and untreated, to respiratory depression occurring secondary to respiratory muscle paralysis (Martin 2003).

The cardiovascular effects of hypermagnesemia can result in ECG changes, which may include prolongation of the PR interval, and widening of the QRS complex. This is due to delayed atrioventricular and interventricular conduction. At severely high serum magnesium levels, complete heart block and asystole can occur. Hypermagnesemia has also been reported to produce hypotension secondary to relaxation of vascular resistance vessels. Myocardial contractility is probably not affected by hypermagnesemia (Martin & Allen-Durrance 2015).

Treatment

Treatment for hypermagnesemia consists importantly in ceasing all exogenous magnesium administration. Any additional treatment is based on the severity of hypermagnesemia, clinical signs observed, and the patient's renal function.

In patients demonstrating only mild clinical signs, they can generally be treated with supportive therapy and observation provided they have normal renal function. In more severe cases, clinical signs can include unresponsiveness and respiratory depression secondary to respiratory muscle paralysis. If patients demonstrate any degree of hemodynamic instability, treatment should include intravenous calcium. Calcium is beneficial in hypermagnesemia as it acts as a direct antagonist at the neuromuscular junction and may reverse the cardiovascular effects arising due to the elevated magnesium levels by stabilizing the threshold potential of the myocardial cells. Calcium gluconate (10% solution) should be given slowly (over 10 minutes) via the intravenous route at a dose rate of 0.5–1.5 mg/kg.

In patients with severe clinical signs, anticholinesterases may also be administered to offset the neurotoxic side effects of hypermagnesemia. Physostigmine can be given at 0.02 mg/kg intravenously every 12 hr until clinical signs subside (Martin & Allen-Durrance 2015). In the most severe cases clinical signs may include cardiopulmonary arrest, in which case intubation and mechanical ventilation are recommended.

References

Bateman, S. W. (2008). Magnesium: A quick reference. *Veterinary Clinics Small Animal Practice* **38**: 467–70.

Bateman, S. W. (2012). Disorders of magnesium: Magnesium deficit and excess. In: S. P. DiBartola (ed.), *Fluid, Electrolyte, and Acid-Base Disorders in Small Animal Practice*, 4th ed. St Louis, MO: W. B. Saunders: 212–229.

Berkelhammer, C. & Bear, R. A. (1985). A clinical approach to common electrolyte problems: 4. Hypomagnesemia. *Canadian Medical Association Journal* **132**: 360–368.

Cortés, Y. E. & Moses, L. (2007). Magnesium disturbances in critically ill patients. *Compendium* **29**(7): 420–427.

Firth, A. (2010). Magnesium: The forgotten ion. *Proceedings of the 16th International Veterinary Emergency and Critical Care Symposium 2010.* San Antonio, TX: 315–317.

Friday, B. A. & Reinhart, R. A. (1990). Magnesium metabolism a case report and literature review. *Critical Care Nurse* **11**: 62–72.

Humphrey, S., Kirby, R., & Rudolf, E. (2015). Magnesium physiology and clinical therapy in veterinary critical care. *Journal of Veterinary Emergency and Critical Care* **25**(2): 210–225.

Jenkinson, D. H. (1957). The nature of the antagonism between calcium and magnesium ions at the neuromuscular junction. *Journal of Physiology* **138**: 434–44.

Martin, L. (2003). Potassium and magnesium and the critically ill. *Proceedings of the 9th International Veterinary Emergency and Critical Care Society,* New Orleans, LA.

Martin, L. G. & Allen-Durrance, A. E. (2015). Magnesium and phosphate disorders. In: D. C. Silverstein & K. Hopper (eds), *Small Animal and Critical Care Medicine.* St Louis, MO: Saunders Elsevier: 281–8.

Martin, L. G., Wingfield, W. E., Van Pelt, D. R., & Hackett, T. B. (1993). Magnesium in the 1990s: Implications for veterinary critical care. *Journal of Veterinary Emergency and Critical Care* **3**(2): 106–14.

Martin, L. G., Matteson, V. L., Wingfield, W. E., et al. (1994). Abnormalities of serum magnesium in critically ill dogs: Incidence and implications. *Journal of Veterinary Emergency and Critical Care* **4**(1 l): 15.

Nakayama, T., Nakayama, H., Miyamoto, M., & Hamlin, R. L. (1999). Hemodynamic and electrocardiographic effects of magnesium sulfate in healthy dogs. *Journal of Veterinary Internal Medicine* **13**(5): 485–90.

Sachter, J. J. (1992). Magnesium in the 1990s: Implications for acute care. *Topics in Emergency Medicine* **14**(1): 23–50.

Whang, R. & Ryder, W. (1990). Frequency of hypomagnesemia and hypermagnesemia. *Journal of the American Medical Association* **263**: 3063–4.

Wingfield, W. E. (2002). Fluid and electrolyte therapy. In: W. E. Wingfield & M. R. Raffe (eds), *The Veterinary ICU Book,* 1st ed. Jackson, WY: Teton New Media: 166–88.

CHAPTER 6

Disorders of Phosphorus

Louise O'Dwyer, MBA BSc (Hons), VTS (Anaesthesia & ECC), DipAVN (Medical & Surgical), RVN

Disorders of phosphorus

Phosphate is the most abundant intracellular anion, and exists in both organic (phospholipids and phosphate esters) and inorganic (orthophosphoric and pyrophosphoric acids) forms and is essential in numerous metabolic processes (e.g. muscle contraction, neuronal impulse conduction, epithelial transport). Strictly speaking, phosphorus is an element and phosphate is a molecular anion (e.g. HPO_4^{2-}), but these terms are often used interchangeably (Martin & Allen-Durrance 2015).

Organic phosphate is present as a constituent in phospholipids, phosphoproteins, nucleic acids, enzymes, adenosine triphosphate (ATP), and cyclic adenosine monophosphate (cAMP). Inorganic phosphate is a substrate in many vital functions of the body, including oxidative phosphorylation, production of 2,3-diphosphoglycerate (2,3-DPG) in erythrocytes (this compound decreases the affinity of hemoglobin for oxygen and facilitates the delivery of oxygen to tissues), and production of glycogen in the liver and kidneys. Phosphorus also stimulates glycolysis by stimulating glycolytic enzymes and participating in phosphorylation of many glycolytic intermediates (Martin 2012).

Phosphate ions play a role in the acid-base balance in serum and in excretion of acids in urine because of their ability to buffer hydrogen ions (H^+) (Forrester & Moreland 1989). Phosphorus in the mammalian body is predominantly (85–90%) present as hydroxyapatite in the mineralized matrix of bone, with most of the remaining (10–15%) occurring in the cytoplasm of cells. Approximately 10–20% of the inorganic phosphate in serum is protein bound, and the remainder circulates as free anion or is complexed to sodium, magnesium, or calcium (DiBartola & Willard 2012). Only a small amount (less than 1%) of non-osseous inorganic phosphate is extracellular and accessible for routine laboratory measurements in

Acid-Base and Electrolyte Handbook for Veterinary Technicians, First Edition.
Edited by Angela Randels-Thorp and David Liss.
© 2017 John Wiley & Sons, Inc. Published 2017 by John Wiley & Sons, Inc.
Companion website: www.wiley.com/go/liss/electrolytes

plasma or serum. Thus, the plasma phosphorus concentration reflects only a small proportion of the total body stores. Depletion of these phosphorus stores is not always reflected in a decrease in the plasma phosphorus concentration. On the other hand, a decreased plasma phosphorus concentration does not always indicate decreased total body phosphorus (Visser 't Hooft, Drobatz, & Ward 2005). Rapid translocations can occur between intracellular and plasma phosphorus pools that can dramatically change the plasma phosphorus concentration. For example, alkalinization of the blood or influx of glucose into cells causes translocation of phosphorus from plasma into cytosol (DiBartola & Willard 2012).

Regulation of phosphorus

Normal serum phosphorus concentrations range from 2.5 to 6.0 mg/dL, but are higher in dogs less than 12 months of age, thereafter they gradually decline. In puppies less than eight weeks of age serum concentrations of up to 10.8 mg/dL may be considered normal. The extent of plasma phosphorus elevation is similar in puppies of giant and small breeds and is approximately 8.5 mg/dL. In cats this effect of age is not as dramatic, but immature animals tend to have higher serum concentrations (DiBartola & Willard 2012). Adult cats tend to have higher mean plasma phosphorus values than adult dogs (Visser 't Hooft, Drobatz, & Ward 2005). Mean plasma phosphorus values in cats younger than 1 year of age are not as elevated as those in young dogs (Chew & Meuten 1982).

Renal function plays a central role in phosphorus metabolism and regulation because phosphorus excretion occurs primarily via the kidneys. Phosphorus is freely filtered by the glomerulus (around 90% of plasma phosphorus) and 80–90% is reabsorbed in the renal tubules. Thus, phosphorus excretion is the net of glomerular filtration less tubular reabsorption of phosphorus. Renal excretion of phosphorus is determined by the glomerular filtration rate (GFR) and the maximum tubular reabsorption rate (Stoff 1982). Most renal phosphorus reabsorption occurs in the proximal convoluted tubule (PCT), with small amounts of phosphorus being reabsorbed in the distal nephron. Reabsorption is sodium dependent because phosphorus transport is performed by a brush border sodium-phosphate co-transporter (Visser 't Hooft, Drobatz, & Ward 2005). Maximal tubular reabsorption of phosphorus can normally be saturated, resulting in phosphaturia when excess phosphorus enters tubular fluid. The regulatory mechanism for renal phosphorus reabsorption can adapt to the body's need for phosphorus through parathyroid hormone (PTH), the major hormonal regulator (DiBartola & Willard 2012). PTH is the most important regulator of renal phosphate transport, as it decreases the tubular transport maximum for phosphate in the proximal tubule where most phosphate reabsorption occurs, whilst at the same time enhancing calcium reabsorption in the distal tubule. Thus, PTH release results in an increased calcium concentration and phosphaturia

(Visser 't Hooft, Drobatz, & Ward 2005). Low blood levels of PTH will result in the opposite effect occurring. The major stimulus for increased PTH synthesis and secretion is a reduced plasma calcium concentration. The major inhibitors of PTH synthesis and secretion are increased concentrations of plasma calcium and 1,25-dihydroxycholecalciferol, the active form of vitamin D (Chew & Meuten 1982). In the presence of phosphorus depletion, the kidneys conserve phosphorus, and the renal response to the phosphaturic effect of PTH is reduced (Visser 't Hooft, Drobatz, & Ward 2005).

Although the kidneys are the major regulator of the plasma phosphorus concentration, the concentration of plasma is ultimately the result of the combined effect of intestinal absorption and excretion, bone resorption and accretion, and renal excretion and reabsorption. The skeleton functions as a reservoir from which phosphorus is mobilized during states of hypophosphatemia. Absorption of dietary phosphorus is approximately 80% and occurs by passive diffusion and by active transport using a sodium-phosphate co-transporter (Visser 't Hooft, Drobatz, & Ward 2005). Absorption occurs in the small intestine, primarily in the mid-jejunum. Because of intestinal phosphorus excretion, a total of about 30–40% of ingested phosphorus is excreted in the feces (Stoff 1982).

The absorption of phosphate in the intestines occurs via two mechanisms: passive diffusion and active mucosal phosphate transport. Passive diffusion is the main route of phosphate absorption, and occurs principally via the paracellular pathway. Active mucosal transport is a sodium-dependent, saturable carrier mediated process (DiBartola & Willard 2012). Calcitriol aids in the process of absorption by increasing intestinal phosphate transport; this system, however, is thought only to be important during dietary phosphate deficiency. These transport mechanisms both function within the duodenum. In the jejunum and ileum the primary process of reabsorption is via diffusion.

Decreased intestinal absorption of phosphorus occurs in vitamin D deficiency, in malabsorption syndromes (e.g. steatorrhea, pancreatitis, lymphangiectasia), and with a phosphorus-deficient diet. In addition, substances containing iron, aluminum (e.g. aluminum hydroxide), or unsaturated fatty acids interfere with intestinal phosphorus absorption (Rosol & Capen 1996). The active form of vitamin D, produced by epithelial cells of the PCTs in the kidneys, increases intestinal absorption of phosphorus and plasma phosphorus concentrations by stimulating bone resorption and possibly by some small contribution of increased renal tubular resorption (Visser 't Hooft, Drobatz, & Ward 2005).

The production of active vitamin D by the kidneys is increased by PTH and a diet low in phosphorus and/or hypophosphatemia (Chew & Meuten 1982). Renal synthesis is also increased by various hormones during growth, pregnancy, and lactation, i.e. growth hormone, estrogen, and prolactin. Renal production of active vitamin D is inhibited by hyperphosphatemia, hypercalcemia, and renal diseases characterized by a loss of renal tubular mass (Rosol & Capen 1996).

Measurement of phosphorus

The majority of phosphate circulates within the body as a free anion but it can be bound to sodium ions (Na^+), magnesium ions ($Mg2^+$), or calcium ions ($Ca2^+$), or to protein (10–15% of total plasma phosphorus; Stoff 1982). Most (80%) plasma inorganic phosphate is in the dibasic form (HPO_4^{2-}) (it is dibasic because it already has one hydrogen so therefore can only accept two more), and the remaining 20% is primarily in the monobasic form (H_2PO^{4-}) (is monobasic since it already has two H^+ ions so can only accept one more), with only a minimal amount as phosphate ions (PO_4^{-3}) (Stoff 1982). This ratio is dependent on the blood pH; at physiologic pH, the average valence to plasma inorganic phosphate is −1.8, indicating that the milliequivalents of plasma phosphorus can be estimated by the following calculation:

1 mmol/L of phosphate = 1.8 mEq/L of phosphate

When alkalemia occurs, more of the dibasic form is present, whereas when acidemia occurs, more monobasic phosphate is present (Lentz, Brown, & Kjellstrand 1978). Therefore, plasma phosphorus levels are usually expressed in milligrams per deciliter for elemental phosphorus or millimoles per liter for phosphate ions because both units, unlike milliequivalents, are independent of the blood pH (3.1 mg of phosphorus/dL = 1 mmol/L of phosphate) (Visser 't Hooft, Drobatz, & Ward 2005).

Whenever measuring phosphorus levels, it should always be borne in mind that plasma phosphorus is an unreliable indicator of body stores: hypophosphatemia does not always imply that phosphorus depletion exists. In contrast, severe phosphorus depletion may be present despite a normal or elevated plasma phosphorus concentration. Phosphorus may rapidly shift between the extracellular and intracellular compartments (Lentz, Brown, & Kjellstrand 1978; Visser 't Hooft, Drobatz, & Ward 2005).

Measurement of phosphorus can be performed using serum or heparinized plasma; citrate, oxalate, or EDTA should not be used as anticoagulants because they interfere with the assay (Visser 't Hooft, Drobatz, & Ward 2005). Fasting blood samples should be taken because a phosphorus-rich meal (e.g. meat) may result in increased plasma phosphorus levels, whereas a carbohydrate-rich meal causes a reduction. It is also important to make every attempt to prevent hemolysis of blood samples, which artificially increases the measurement because of release of intracellular stores of inorganic phosphate. To prevent leakage of cellular phosphorus, serum or plasma should be separated from cells within 1 hr of collection (Stoff 1982; Bourke & Yanagawa 1993). Plasma calcium and phosphorus values should be evaluated concurrently because their normal regulation and control are so interrelated (see Chapter 7 on calcium). False decreases in plasma phosphorus concentrations may also be seen with hyperbilirubinemia or hyperlipidemia. This occurs because of interference with the colorimetric determination (Bourke & Yanagawa 1993). There have also been reports of pseudo-hypophosphatemia, a 1998 study by Harkin et al. found this to occur in two dogs with icterus and hemolysis because of immune-mediated hemolytic anemia.

Hypophosphatemia

Whenever hypophosphatemia is encountered, it should be remembered that blood chemistry analyzers will not necessarily reflect whole body phosphate balance, due to the rapid shifts that can occur from the extracellular to the intracellular space. Normal ranges of phosphate are 2.9–5.3 mg/dL (dependent upon the patient's age and the individual biochemistry analyzer) (Martin 2012). In cases of mild to moderate hypophosphatemia (1.0–2.5 mg/dL), such levels may not be concerning, and may not necessarily be associated with phosphate depletion, dependent on the individual patient and their clinical signs. However, once levels are < 1 mg/dL (severe hypophosphatemia), this is generally a clinically significant level and tends to be associated with a total body phosphate depletion, but again individual patient assessment is required.

Causes

There are a number of causes of hypophosphatemia, including decreased intestinal absorption, increased renal phosphorus loss (including increased urinary excretion), and transcellular shift of phosphorus from the blood into cells (Knochel 1977). See Table 6.1.

As discussed, the translocation of inorganic phosphorus from the extracellular fluid to intracellular locations can occur rapidly and significantly decrease plasma phosphorus levels. This can be caused by increased insulin levels (e.g. insulin administration, intravenous infusions of glucose, feeding high-carbohydrate diets). Insulin promotes intracellular uptake of phosphorus needed for increased glycolysis and phosphorylation of ADP to ATP. Rapid repair and regeneration of damaged tissue may cause uptake of extracellular phosphorus, resulting in hypophosphatemia (Visser 't Hooft, Drobatz, & Ward 2005).

Much of the discussion about hypophosphatemia in the veterinary literature tends to be related to diabetes mellitus; hypophosphatemia can be common in diabetic ketoacidosis, as a result of excess phosphorus loss via the urine. This arises due to polyuria (i.e. an osmotic diuresis) and because of decreased tubular reabsorption of phosphorus due to the presence of glucose and ketones in the tubular fluid (Visser 't Hooft, Drobatz, & Ward 2005). This process can be worsened because of metabolic acidosis, which enhances phosphaturia as a result of intracellular organic phosphate compound, which causes the phosphorus to move into the plasma, and then is excreted via the urine (Knochel 1977). In patients that are anorexic, or vomiting, a concurrent decrease in phosphorus can also occur.

Table 6.1 Causes of hypophosphatemia (Source: Based on data from Martin 2012: 285)

Decreased Gastrointestinal Absorption	Transcellular shifts	Increased renal/urinary loss	Spurious/lab error
Chronic malnutrition	Alkalosis (respiratory or metabolic)	A) Diuresis 1 Osmotic • Diabetes mellitus/diabetic ketoacidosis • Hyperosmolar hyperglycemic non-ketotic syndrome • Recovery phase of third degree burns 2 Drug induced • Carbonic anhydrase inhibitors • Mannitol 3 Post-obstructive 4 Hypothermia induced 5 Parenteral fluid therapy	A) Monoclonal gammopathy B) Hemolysis C) Hyperbilirubinemia D) Mannitol (blood levels > 25 mmol/L)
Malabsorptive syndromes	Intravenous dextrose administration	B) Hyperparathyroidism 1 Primary 2 Secondary	
Steatorrhea	Insulin therapy	C) Hyperaldosteronism	
Chronic vomiting and/or diarrhea	Refeeding syndrome	D) Glucocorticoid therapy with or without hyperadrenocorticism	
Vitamin D deficiency	Catecholamines (endogenous or exogenous)	E) Parenteral fluid therapy	
Phosphate binding antacids	Salicylate poisoning		
	Eclampsia		
	Hypercalcemia of malignancy		

On presentation, even though these patients may have actual phosphorus depletion, their plasma phosphorus concentrations can still be normal, or even elevated, as a result of both insulin deficiency and metabolic acidosis, which can result in a shift of phosphorus out of the cells (Kebler, McDonald, & Cadnapaphornchai 1985). Once treatment presents in these patients, i.e. insulin administration, this transcellular shift can be reversed, and the plasma phosphorus concentration can rapidly decline. This will promote phosphorus (and glucose) entry into the cells under the influence of the enzyme hexokinase. Insulin and glucose stimulate glycolysis, promoting the synthesis of phosphorylated glucose compounds and intracellular shifts of phosphate. This can result in the aggravation of the existing hypophosphatemia, or can result in the onset of hypophosphatemia as a new clinical problem. Hypophosphatemia becomes evident in the first 24 hr following insulin therapy and peaks in severity within 24–36 hr (Visser 't Hooft, Drobatz, & Ward 2005).

Hyperventilation causes respiratory alkalosis, which will lead to a rapid diffusion of carbon dioxide from the intracellular space to the extracellular space. The increase in intracellular pH activates phosphofructokinase and glycolysis, resulting in phosphate shifting rapidly into the cells (Martin 2012). Respiratory alkalosis can occur as a result of fear, pain, septicemia, and central nervous system disorders (e.g. seizures).

Hypophosphatemia as a result of refeeding syndrome has long been identified and is well published in human medicine and is now also an important topic in veterinary medicine. Long-standing starvation or a poor nutritional status may deplete intracellular phosphorus pools but rarely leads to hypophosphatemia. If diets used to reverse the catabolic state in these patients are low in phosphorus, hypophosphatemia may result from transcellular shifts of phosphorus and glucose into cells. This is particularly important when refeeding cats with anorexia-induced hepatic lipidosis, or increased alanine aminotransferase activity, hyperbilirubinemia, and weight loss may result in a syndrome similar to the starvation/refeeding syndrome described in humans (Adams et al. 1993). It is also thought that calcium may also play a role in phosphorus losses in animals during the early stages of starvation and in association with total parenteral nutrition (Visser 't Hooft, Drobatz, & Ward 2005).

Hypovitaminosis D as a cause of decreased gastrointestinal absorption is often cited as a cause of hypophosphatemia, but this alone is an unlikely cause of low plasma phosphorus levels, but it may be contributory. Vitamin D deficiency can arise because of a lack of exposure to sunlight, inadequate amounts of vitamin D in the diet, or steatorrhea, which results in intestinal malabsorption of vitamin D (Knochel & Jacobson 1986). If overused, gastrointestinal protectants and antacids containing aluminum hydroxide or magnesium hydroxide may combine with phosphorus, thereby limiting its absorption from the intestine.

Hypophosphatemia can also arise because of increased renal excretion of phosphorus. PTH is a phosphaturic hormone; therefore, either primary or nutritional secondary hyperparathyroidism may result in hypophosphatemia. Primary hyper-aldosteronism can result in renal loss of calcium, resulting in hypocalcaemia, which, in turn, stimulates secretion of PTH and may result in normal or low serum phosphate.

Primary hyperparathyroidism and pseudohyperparathyroidism result in increased circulating plasma PTH or PTH-related protein levels, which enhance phosphaturia. Hypercalcemia has a direct effect on tubular cells, which enhances phosphaturia, thereby contributing to the development of hypophosphatemia. If renal function is impaired, this situation may not occur and therefore hypophosphatemia might not be present. Renal secondary hyperparathyroidism is stimulated by transient or persistent elevations of plasma phosphorus levels as a result of a decreased GFR. Thus, this condition is not associated with hypophosphatemia (Visser 't Hooft, Drobatz, & Ward 2005).

Clinical signs

The clinical signs of hypophosphatemia in small animals can be very varied, with many severely hypophosphatemic patients not actually demonstrating any clinical signs of hypophosphatemia. Phosphorus is an important component of ATP and is therefore critical in certain energy-dependent physiologic processes. ATP is also required to maintain the integrity of cell membranes and cell shape and deformability. Therefore, depletion of ATP and 2,3-DPG is the cause of many of the severe clinical signs associated with hypophosphatemia. This means nearly every organ system susceptible to the effects of hypophosphatemia. Hypophosphatemia mainly affects body cells that are high-energy users, including erythrocytes, skeletal muscle cells, and brain cells. Intracellular inorganic phosphate is a cofactor in anaerobic glycolysis, the sole pathway for erythrocyte synthesis of ATP and 2,3-DPG (Visser 't Hooft, Drobatz, & Ward 2005). In erythrocytes, the lack of ATP and decreased production of intracellular 2,3-DPG can cause both structural and functional abnormalities (Kono, Kuwajima, & Turai 1981). Decreased 2,3-DPG increases the affinity of hemoglobin for oxygen. This causes a left shift of the oxyhemoglobin dissociation curve; this results in impaired oxygen delivery to peripheral tissues. Subsequent hypoxia is thought to be the cause of many of the clinical manifestations of hypophosphatemia (Knochel 1977).

Hemolysis is the most common complication of hypophosphatemia (Adams et al. 1993). Hemolysis occurs because of depleted ATP levels in erythrocytes, with the concentration of erythrocyte ATP correlating closely with membrane deform ability. In experimental models in dogs, hemolysis was induced only at very low plasma phosphorus concentrations (i.e. <0.5 mg/dL). However, cats may be more sensitive than other species because hypophosphatemia-induced hemolysis has been described in cats with plasma phosphorus concentrations of above 1 mg/dL. In hemolytic cases, a decrease in hematocrit was seen within 24–48 hr after documented hypophosphatemia (Adams et al. 1993; Visser 't Hooft, Drobatz, & Ward 2005).

Severe hypophosphatemia can also impair leukocyte function secondary to depletion of cellular ATP. Leukocytes may show impaired chemotaxis, phagocytosis, and intracellular killing functions, making patients more susceptible to infection (Yawata et al. 1974). In addition, to the effects on leukocytes and erythrocytes, platelets may function poorly, resulting in impaired clot retraction and cutaneous hemorrhage, and a decreased platelet survival time in the blood. Thrombocytopenia and large-diameter platelets have been observed (Adams et al. 1993; Yawata et al. 1974).

Severe hypophosphatemia has been associated with myocardial dysfunction in humans and is a proposed mechanism for cardiac dysrhythmias (Martin 2012). Severe hypophosphatemia may impair myocardial performance by reducing the energy-generating ability of the left ventricle. In a study of hypophosphatemia (0.9 mg/dL) in phosphorus-deprived dogs, they found decreased myocardial stroke volume independent of the Frank-Starling effect. Dietary phosphorus repletion resulted in rapid resolution of cardiac abnormalities. The myocardial consequences of severe hypophosphatemia are thought to result from depleted intracellular ATP stores and/or impaired calcium metabolism (Fuller et al. 1978).

Moderate hypophosphatemia can result in a proximal myopathy characterized by weakness, osteomalacia, bone pain, muscle atrophy, and normal plasma activity of creatinine kinase (Visser 't Hooft, Drobatz, & Ward 2005). These abnormalities are reversible with phosphorus repletion. Acute, severe hypophosphatemia can cause generalized myopathy characterized by muscle necrosis (rhabdomyolysis), myoglobinuria, diffuse muscle pain, generalized weakness, and elevated creatine kinase values (Adams et al. 1993). In the most severe cases hypophosphatemia has been associated with ataxia, convulsions, stupor, and death (Visser 't Hooft, Drobatz, & Ward 2005).

Treatment

Most cases of hypophosphatemia do not require specific treatment. A positive outcome can be achieved by successfully managing the underlying condition(s) detected, normalizing a patient's acid-base status, and resuming a normal diet. This treatment protocol will generally result in returning plasma phosphorus levels to normal.

A variety of oral phosphorus supplements are available in the form of sodium, potassium, and calcium phosphate salts. Oral supplementation is safer and thus preferable to parenteral supplementation, but dosing in veterinary medicine is empiric. For adult dogs, the phosphorus requirement is estimated to be 1.4–4.6 g/1000 kcal of metabolizable energy; for adult cats, the estimated requirement is 1.25 g/1000 kcal of metabolizable energy (Visser 't Hooft, Drobatz, & Ward 2005). Oral phosphorus supplements should be used cautiously as they can cause diarrhea and therefore should be given in multiple small doses.

In cases of severe hypophosphatemia intravenous phosphorus administration is warranted, rather than oral phosphorus supplementation (Stoff 1982).

Intravenous therapy may also be required when oral intake is precluded by anorexia, vomiting, altered consciousness, or inability to absorb phosphorus from the intestine (Visser 't Hooft, Drobatz, & Ward 2005). Parenteral supplementation is available in the form of potassium phosphate and sodium phosphate.

Because many severely hypophosphatemic patients have concurrent hypokalemia, potassium phosphate solution is maybe most appropriate as a therapeutic agent. Potassium phosphate (KH_2PO_4) solution contains 4.36–4.4 mEq/ml of potassium and 3 mmol/ml (99.1 mg/ml) of phosphate (Visser 't Hooft, Drobatz, & Ward 2005; Martin 2014). Sodium phosphate solution (Na_2HPO_4) contains 4 mEq/ml of sodium and 3 mmol/ml (93 mg/ml) of phosphate (Adams et al. 1993, Martin 2014). It should be remembered that both potassium phosphate and sodium phosphate solutions are hypertonic and therefore require dilution before use. They should be administered in calcium-free fluids, such as 0.9% saline or 5% dextrose solutions, to prevent precipitation of insoluble calcium phosphate salts (Adams et al. 1993). It is also vitally important to account for the total amount of potassium being supplemented as part of the patient's fluid therapy plan, in order to avoid accidental hyperkalemia.

Individual patient's phosphorus requirements are highly variable and very much dependent on the underlying cause, duration, and pathogenesis of hypophosphatemia and plasma phosphorus concentration is an unreliable indicator of total body stores. Careful monitoring of clinical efficacy and plasma phosphorus concentrations can aid in making dosage adjustments. The recommended dose is 0.01–0.03 mmol/kg/hr of intravenous phosphate infusion for 6 hr until the plasma phosphorus level is more than 2 mg/dL (Visser 't Hooft, Drobatz, & Ward 2005). During parenteral administration of phosphorus, plasma phosphorus concentration should be monitored every 3–6 hr. The dosage should subsequently be adjusted according to the results of plasma phosphorus determinations. In most cases, two to four treatments of potassium phosphate at 6 hr intervals were necessary to increase the phosphorus concentration to more than 2.5 mg/dL (Visser 't Hooft, Drobatz, & Ward 2005). The plasma phosphorus concentration should be monitored continually to assess the efficacy of therapy and prevent hypophosphatemia, even after return to normophosphatemia. The potential adverse effects of rapid phosphorus supplementation include hyperphosphatemia, hypocalcemia, with associated tetany, metastatic calcification, and renal failure (Martin 2014).

Hyperphosphatemia

Elevated phosphorus levels in a veterinary patient may, or may not, be termed hyperphosphatemia, depending on the age of the animal. As already stated, normal serum phosphate levels are between 2.9 and 5.3 mg/dL, but concentrations up to 10 mg/dL have been reported in healthy puppies (Martin 2014).

Causes

Hyperphosphatemia can result from decreased renal excretion, hypervitaminosis D, hypoparathyroidism, increased phosphorus intake, or iatrogenic administration, and transcellular shifts/translocation (acute tumor lysis syndrome). In veterinary medicine the most commonly cited cause of hyperphosphatemia is reduced renal excretion as a result of acute kidney injury (AKI) or chronic kidney disease (CKD) (Yawata et al. 1974; Schropp & Kovacic 2007). Hyperphosphatemia results in the inhibition of 1α–hydroxylase activity and stimulates the secretion of PTH.

Chronic renal failure

Decreased renal function results in an alteration of calcium/phosphate homeostasis. In the early stages, there is decreased serum calcitriol and decreased calcium levels which result in the increased synthesis of PTH. Later, decreased vitamin D and calcium receptors contribute to further increase of PTH. Increased PTH leads to decreased phosphate excretion, increased dietary phosphate retention and increased serum phosphate levels. Increased serum phosphate will lead to further PTH synthesis. This condition is known as secondary hyperparathyroidism (Schropp & Kovacic 2007).

Iatrogenic toxicities

Hyperphosphatemia can occasionally be observed in patients following the administration of phosphate-containing enemas. Clinical signs seen include severe dehydration and electrolyte disorders, which, if severe enough, can result in death. The ingestion of vitamin D3 containing skin preparations used for psoriasis (e.g. calcipotriene) can result in acute severe hypercalcemia, hyperphosphatemia, and widespread tissue mineralization. The ingestion of certain rodenticides (e.g. those containing cholecalciferol) can also cause similar effects within 12–36 hr of ingestion, and despite treatment may be fatal (Murphy 2002). Iatrogenic overdose due to ingestion of large volumes of phosphorus supplements or urinary acidifiers can also occur (Schropp & Kovacic 2007).

Acute tumor-lysis syndrome

Acute tumor-lysis syndrome can be observed in patients within around 48 hr following the administration of their first chemotherapy treatment. It is more commonly seen in patients under treatment for highly responsive lymphoma, and occurs as a result of cell destruction, which results in massive release of potassium and phosphate. Patients receiving chemotherapy for cancers such as stage IV or V lymphoma with a large tumor burden are most at risk for acute tumor-lysis syndrome, especially if already volume depleted and azotemic (Ogilvie 2004).

Hypoparathyroidism

A less common cause of hyperphosphatemia is hypoparathyroidism. This condition is commonly diagnosed when the patient presents with neuromuscular symptoms secondary to hypocalcemia. The underlying cause of hypoparathyroidism is a PTH deficiency, and patients may present with a variety of symptoms, including restlessness, weakness, and ataxia progressing to acute seizures or tetany. An initial diagnosis of hypoparathyroidism is made based on the patient's clinical signs, hypocalcaemia, and hyperphosphatemia with normal renal values. Acute treatment includes calcium supplementation and vitamin D therapy for long-term management (Schropp & Kovacic 2007).

Clinical signs

Patients with hypoparathyroidism typically present with clinical signs of hyperphosphatemia and hypocalcemia, including: anorexia, nausea, vomiting, weakness, tetany, seizures, and arrhythmias (Martin 2014). Hyperphosphatemia often occurs alongside hypocalcaemia, hypomagnesaemia, hypernatremia, and metabolic acidosis, with the clinical manifestations often arising due to hypercalcemia and metastatic soft tissue calcification.

Treatment

Treatment of hyperphosphatemia involves administration of dextrose containing intravenous fluids (crystalloids) that will correct any underlying acidosis, increase intracellular uptake of phosphate, resolve azotemia, and correct calcium imbalances (Schropp & Kovacic 2007). The ultimate goal of treatment is the treatment of the underlying disorder. In cases of chronic renal failure, the use of phosphate binders may be required because improvement of renal function may not be achievable.

References

Adams, L. G., Hardy, R. M., Weiss, D. J., & Bartges, J. W. (1993). Hypophosphatemia and hemolytic anemia associated with diabetes mellitus and hepatic lipidosis in cats. *Journal of Veterinary Internal Medicine* **7**(5): 266–71.

Bourke, E. & Yanagawa, N. (1993). Assessment of hyperphosphatemia and hypophosphatemia. *Clinical Laboratory Medicine* **13**: 183–205.

Chew, D. J. & Meuten, D. J. (1982). Disorders of calcium and phosphorus metabolism. *Veterinary Clinics of North America Small Animal Practice* **12**(3): 411–438.

DiBartola, S. P. & Willard, M. D. (2012). Disorders of phosphorus: Hypophosphatemia and hyperphosphatemia. In: S. P. DiBartola (ed.), *Fluid Therapy in Small Animal Practice*. Philadelphia, W. B. Saunders: 163–74.

Forrester, S. D. & Moreland, K. J. (1989). Hypophosphatemia: Causes and clinical consequences. *Journal of Veterinary Internal Medicine* **3**:149–159.

Fuller, T. J., Nichols, W. W., Brenner, B. J., & Peterson, J. C. (1978). Reversible depression in myocardial performance in dogs with experimental phosphorus deficiency. *Journal of Clinical Investigation* **62**: 1194–200.

Harkin, K. R., Braselton, W. E., & Tvedten, H. (1998). Pseudohypophosphatemia in two dogs with immune-mediated hemolytic anemia. *Journal of Veterinary Internal Medicine* **12**:178–81.

Kebler, R., McDonald, F. D., & Cadnapaphornchai, P. (1985). Dynamic changes in serum phosphorus levels in diabetic ketoacidosis. *American Journal of Medicine* **79**:571–6.

Knochel, J. P. (1977). The pathophysiology and clinical characteristics of severe hypophosphatemia. *Archives of Internal Medicine* **137**: 203–20.

Knochel, J. P. & Jacobson, H. R. (1986). Renal handling of phosphorus, clinical hypophosphatemia, and phosphorus deficiency. In: B. M. Brenner & F. C. Rector (eds), *The Kidney*. Philadelphia, W. B. Saunders: 619–662.

Kono, N., Kuwajima, M., & Turai, S. (1981). Alteration of glycolytic intermediary metabolism in erythrocytes during diabetic ketoacidosis and its recovery phase. *Diabetes* **30**: 346.

Lentz, R. D., Brown, D. M., & Kjellstrand, C. M. (1978). Treatment of severe hypophosphatemia. *Annals of Internal Medicine* **89**: 941–4.

Martin, L. (2012). Magnesium and phosphate disorders In: D. C. Silverstein & K. Hopper (eds), *Small Animal Critical Care Medicine*. St Louis, MO: Saunders Elsevier: 281–88.

Martin, L. G. & Allen-Durrance, A. E. (2015). Magnesium and phosphate disorders. In D. C. Silverstein & K. Hopper (eds), *Small Animal and Critical Care Medicine*. St Louis, MO: Saunders Elsevier: 281–8.

Murphy, M. J. (2002). Rodenticides. *Veterinary Clinics of North America Small Animal Practice* **32**(2): 469–84.

Ogilvie, G. K. (2004). Red alert! Rapid response to the collapsed or seizuring cancer patient. *International Veterinary Emergency and Critical Care Symposium 2004 Proceedings*, San Diego, CA.

Rosol, T. J. & Capen, C. C. (1996). Pathophysiology of calcium, phosphorus, and magnesium metabolism in animals. *Veterinary Clinics of North America Small Animal Practice* **26**(5): 1155–82.

Schropp, D. M. & Kovacic, J. (2007). Phosphorus and phosphate metabolism in veterinary patients. *Journal of Veterinary Emergency and Critical Care* **17**(2): 127–34.

Stoff, J. S. (1982). Phosphate homeostasis and hypophosphatemia. *American Journal of Medicine* **72**:489–95.

Visser 't Hooft, K., Drobatz, K. J., & Ward, C. R. (2005). Hypophosphatemia. *Compendium* December: 900–911.

Yawata, Y., Hebbel, R. P., Silvis, S., et al. (1974). Blood cell abnormalities complicating the hypophosphatemia of hyperalimentation: Erythrocyte and platelet ATP deficiency associated with hemolytic anemia and bleeding in hyperalimented dogs. *Journal of Laboratory and Clinical Medicine* **84**: 643–53.

CHAPTER 7

Disorders of Calcium

Katherine Howie, RVN, VTS (ECC)

Physiology of calcium

The normal physiology of calcium is tightly regulated and requires synergistic actions from calcium regulatory hormones to ensure that calcium homeostasis remains controlled. Variations of calcium outside of the narrow range needed to carry out vital intracellular and extracellular functions can lead to damage at cellular level, tissue level or potentially affect entire body systems. Calcium is a major contributor to cellular energy provision and as such homeostasis is essential.

The primary source of calcium intake is dietary and enteric absorption will be dependent upon the health of the gastrointestinal tract (GIT) as well as vitamin D synthesis. As well as calcium, which is required as part of a balanced diet, our small animal patients also require vitamin D to be provided at suitable levels. As they are unable to synthesize vitamin D in the skin, it needs to be provided in the diet for enteric absorption and then metabolism to the active metabolites that assist with the regulation of calcium. Normal dietary requirements of calcium will be 100 mg/kg with between 10–35 mg/kg being absorbed for use. Once calcium has been absorbed from the GIT, it will present in the extracellular fluid (ECF). From there it can be absorbed into the soft tissue, the skeletal system or excreted via urine or feces (Hazewinkel 1991).

As we can see from this, the absorption will depend upon the amount of calcium in the diet being appropriate for the life stage of the animal and providing the correct amount of dietary calcium and vitamin D for absorption. There is perhaps more of a concern now with the advent of raw meat diets and homemade diets that there may be inappropriate levels of calcium and other vitamins and minerals for appropriate intake and absorption; as such, this should be explored with the client when addressing primary dietary disorders of calcium.

Acid-Base and Electrolyte Handbook for Veterinary Technicians, First Edition.
Edited by Angela Randels-Thorp and David Liss.
© 2017 John Wiley & Sons, Inc. Published 2017 by John Wiley & Sons, Inc.
Companion website: www.wiley.com/go/liss/electrolytes

A fully balanced homemade diet should not cause significant problems; however, there is a high risk of these diets not being balanced with inappropriate calcium:phosphorous ratios and unsuitable quantities of vitamin D, all of which are necessary for appropriate absorption and utilization of dietary calcium (Freeman et al. 2013).

Abnormal serum concentrations of calcium are important even if they are only slightly deviated from normal as the regulation and room for deviations in calcium can lead to detrimental clinical signs in our patients. While a high or low serum calcium does not give a diagnosis, it can be indicative of many acute or chronic disease states. It is also important to remember that a patient may have disruption of the homeostatic mechanisms that maintain calcium but have a normal serum ionized calcium. Calcium at a cellular level provides energy for the adenosine triphosphate (ATP) pump via the calcium channels; as such, any intra- or extracellular shifts of calcium may result in failure of the ATP pump and influx of sodium and calcium ions into the intracellular space, leading to cellular swelling, damage, or death.

The homeostatic mechanisms that control calcium retention and excretion allow the body only to store what is required and excretes the remainder to avoid hypocalcemic and hypercalcemic states in a healthy patient. Normal calcium balance in the small animal patient is regulated by the parathyroid hormone (PTH), vitamin D metabolites, and calcitonin. PTH is responsible for minute-by-minute responses to changes in calcium, whereas calcitonin acts over a longer period and is responsible for day-to-day changes in calcium levels within the body. When we consider calcium and alterations in the homeostatic mechanisms, it is important to know how calcium is stored and excreted within the body. These storage mechanisms play a vital role in homeostatic control; as such, any disruption in the body's systems affected by calcium regulatory hormones or the cells where these hormones act can cause disruption of storage and excretion and alterations of serum calcium levels. Also any disease process that affects the production of PTH, metabolism of vitamin D, or calcitonin levels may affect the homeostatic mechanisms involved. See Figure 7.1.

The main organs affected by the calcium regulatory hormones are the intestine (responsible for absorption and excretion), the kidneys (also responsible for excretion), and the bone (responsible for absorption and mobilization of calcium in response to acute changes of calcium levels).

When the gastrointestinal or renal absorption mechanisms are affected by a disease state, the skeletal system will provide a major supply of calcium and phosphorous in the short term by mobilizing calcium and to a lesser degree phosphorous from storage within the skeletal system.

Almost all (99%) of body calcium is stored as hydroxyapatite, $Ca_{10}(PO_4)_6(OH)_2$ and resides in the skeleton. Most skeletal calcium is poorly exchangeable or bioavailable with less than 1% considered bioavailable. Any amount that is considered rapidly available is a result of ECF in bone, which is present between the

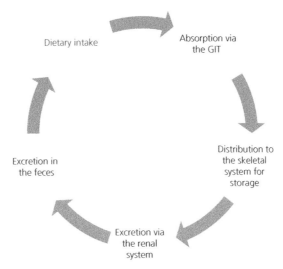

Figure 7.1 Body systems responsible for calcium regulation.

osteoblasts, osteocytes, and bone matrix. The large majority of non-skeletal calcium is maintained within the ECF; however, small but important quantities are available in the intracellular fluid (ICF), which can be transported by proteins out of the intracellular space (Rosol et al. 1995; Schenck & Chew 2005; Schenck, Chew, & Behrend 2006).

Extracellular calcium concentrations should be considered alongside the "type" of calcium and the bioavailability in plasma or serum. Ionized calcium accounts for approximately 56%; this is perhaps the most important as it is a biologically active and therefore available for use within the serum. Other sources of extracellular calcium include that which is protein bound which accounts for approximately 35% of calcium in ECF (Schenck, Chew, & Brooks 1996). Although there is a significant percentage of calcium bound to proteins, the actual role of protein with calcium is simply as a storage or buffering system for ionized calcium—no other biological role has been discovered. Complexed calcium is that which is bound to phosphate, bicarbonate, sulfate, citrate, and lactate and accounts for approximately 10% of serum total calcium concentration (Schenck, Chew, & Brooks 1996).

Intracellular calcium is maintained in a normal patient at a very low level. It is an important secondary messenger through the cell membrane and responds to biochemical signals. At a low level in a normal patient it assists with cellular function transport of ions into and out of the intracellular space alongside other vital functions. If intracellular calcium levels are not maintained at a low level, this can lead to cell toxicity and cellular death due to the toxic effects of high levels of calcium in the intracellular space and reduced excitability of cellular membranes (Rosol et al. 1995; Rasmussen et al. 1990). Calcium within the body plays an essential role in coagulation, muscle contraction, neural excitability, hormone release, and membrane permeability. Storage, excretion, and absorption of calcium are all important and are regulated by the calcium regulatory hormones. Due to the diverse nature of the roles calcium plays within the body to maintain homeostasis in many different tissues, muscles, and organ systems, there will be thousands of different functions relying on suitable control at any one time.

Parathyroid hormone is produced within the chief cells of the parathyroid gland and controlled and synthesized by feedback on the serum levels of calcium and to a lesser degree magnesium. PTH has a short half-life of 3–5 minutes in serum and as such a constant low rate of secretion is normally required to maintain serum PTH levels. PTH is normally secreted at around 25% of the maximum rate and is secreted steadily in normocalcemia (Kronenberg et al. 2001). The stimulus for an increase in PTH secretion is hypocalcemia. The primary function of PTH is to control calcium concentration in the ECF, which it does by affecting the rate of transfer of calcium into and out of bone, resorption in the kidneys via the renal tubules, and absorption from the GIT. The effect on the kidneys is the most rapid, causing reabsorption of calcium and excretion of phosphorus. The initial effect of PTH on bone is to mobilize calcium into the ECF. Small amounts of PTH are stored within the parathyroid gland, and as such synthesis, secretion, and decreasing the amount of PTH released are all controlled by the chief cells in the parathyroid gland. The parathyroid cell processes are controlled by calcitriol via the vitamin D receptor and extracellular iCa concentration exerting an effect at the plasmalemmel calcium receptor. Calcitriol exerts overall control on PTH synthesis and secretion, because it regulates expression of the calcium receptor gene. Intact PTH molecules are destroyed by phagocytosis as well as fragments of degraded PTH being filtered by the renal system (DiBartola 2012; Massry & Glassock 2001; Patel et al. 1995).

Vitamin D (calciferol) is considered to be a major hormone related to the control of intracellular and extracellular calcium levels. The term "vitamin" when considering calciferol and the metabolites cholecalciferol or ergocalciferol is imprecise when discussing the many functions of vitamin D. Dogs and cats are unable to synthesize vitamin D3 (cholecalciferol) in the skin and depend upon appropriate dietary intake. Again, as mentioned previously, there is a concern with more clients making homemade diets that vitamin D is provided at inappropriate levels and this can subsequently lead to inappropriate levels of vitamin D and regulatory problems in the calcium homeostatic mechanisms due to low vitamin D levels or excessive provision of vitamin D in the diet. If a patient has a high intake of dietary vitamin D, there is the potential for toxicity to arise (Freeman et al. 2013). There are around 30 metabolites of vitamin D; however, only three are considered relevant when discussing calcium absorption and excretion. Vitamin D must be metabolically activated before it can function physiologically, meaning any vitamin D ingested in the diet must undergo metabolism or hydroxylation before it can be involved in the homeostatic mechanisms for absorption of calcium. The mechanism of metabolism for vitamin D is reliant upon the patient receiving enough vitamin D within the diet and vitamin D being absorbed as a whole from the intestine before being metabolized. Once the molecule is ingested, it is transported by binding proteins to the hepatic system and other target cells and sites. Vitamin D needs to be metabolized to a certain degree in the liver by the process of hydroxylation, which produces calcidol—one of the metabolites of vitamin D. The next, and most limiting, step in metabolism is the further metabolism of calcidol to calcitriol within the renal tubule. Synthesis of PTH, calcitriol, phosphorous, and calcium are the main regulators for calcitriol synthesis via the renal tubules. This conversion in the kidneys is the rate-limiting step in vitamin D metabolism, and as such we may see a delay in the bioavailability of vitamin D once it has been administered therapeutically. PTH and conditions that stimulate its secretion, as well as hypophosphatemia, increase the formation of the active vitamin D metabolite. It would be expected that there would be an increase in secretion and synthesis of vitamin D metabolites during pregnancy, lactation, and growth. Vitamin D metabolites that remain unchanged are excreted in bile and subsequently the feces (Bowen 2011).

Calcitriol is recognized to be the only natural form of vitamin D with significant biological activity (Deluca, Krisinger, & Darwish 1990). Calcitriol stimulates resorption of calcium and phosphorous from the kidney as well as having an effect in the intestine. Calcitriol actions include indirect effects on calcium balance, including upregulation of calcitriol receptors in patients with renal failure and associated uremia, a role in regulation of PTH synthesis and secretion (Galvao et al. 2013), and limiting or reversing parathyroid gland hyperplasia in the uremic patient (Deluca, Krisinger, & Darwish 1990; Galvao et al. 2013).

The effects of calcitriol include all of the following:

- enhanced transport of calcium and phosphate from the lumen of the GIT into plasma via the enterocytes (Bronner 2003; Wasserman 1981);
- induces synthesis of the ATP pump allowing energy to be created and calcium to be transported across the enterocytes into the ECF;
- calcitriol is also essential in the formation and mineralization of bone due to its effects on the GIT and absorption of calcium and phosphorous, which is essential for skeletal health (Bowen 2011);
- calcitriol is required to work in synergy with PTH to resorb calcium from the urinary system into blood;
- calcitriol is considered to protect the kidneys in chronic renal failure from excessive amounts of PTH but is also being considered as having beneficial effects on the diseased kidney (Nagode, Chew, & Steinmeyer 1992);
- calcitriol can inhibit PTH synthesis by binding to its specific receptors in the parathyroid chief cells (Nagode, Chew, & Steinmeyer 1992);
- due to the fact calcitriol stimulates intestinal calcium absorption, it can also reduce PTH secretion by increasing ionized calcium levels—suppression of PTH synthesis cannot occur without the presence of calcitriol even if there is hypercalcemia (Nagode, Chew, & Steinmeyer 1992; Nagode, Chew, & Podell 1996);

- calcitriol has been discussed as a treatment therapy for patients in early stages of chronic renal failure to avoid hyperparathyroidism (Nagode, Chew, & Steinmeyer 1992; Nagode, Chew, & Podell 1996).

Calcitonin is secreted by the parafollicular cells, or C cells, in the thyroid gland. Secretion of calcitonin by the C cells reduces the concentration of calcium ions in the ECF and is a regulatory response in the face of hypercalcemia (Ettinger & Feldman 2010). Calcitonin interacts with target cells primarily within the bone and kidney (responsible for storage and release in the case of bone and excretion in the case of the kidney), and the actions of parathyroid hormone and calcitonin are synergistic in reducing renal tubular absorption of phosphorous. Hypophosphatemia develops from a direct action of calcitonin, which inhibits bone resorption and increases the rate of movement of phosphorous out of plasma into soft tissues and bones by inhibiting bone resorption stimulated by PTH and other factors. The effects of calcitonin in the face of hyper- or hypocalcemia are considered minor (Schenck et al. 2012: 134).

Another ion that is closely interrelated with calcium specifically is phosphorous. Calcium and phosphorous are closely associated with each other in animal metabolism. Adequate calcium and phosphorous nutrition depends on: a sufficient supply of each nutrient, a suitable ratio between them, and the presence of vitamin D. These three factors are interrelated. A suitable calcium:phosphorous ratio would be considered 1:1 or 2:1 and vitamin D is essential for utilization (Barrette 1988). The relationship between calcium and phosphorus is discussed in Chapter 6.

Normal factors affecting phosphorous storage and excretion may be compromised in renal failure, which is why we can subsequently see patients in chronic renal failure with not only elevated serum phosphorous levels and hypo- or hypercalcemia but also changes to the structure, density, and function of the bone in patients with chronic renal failure due to the regulatory hormones and storage mechanisms being affected.

Calcium is released from the bone matrix and ECF and travels through the circulation either bound to proteins such as albumin or as free ions attached to minerals which can then be transported intracellularly to act as secondary messengers playing an important role in signal conduction pathways, neurotransmitter release from neurons, and contraction of all muscle types. Additionally, calcium ions are required as co-factors for enzymes within the coagulation cascade, for example. These ions are also utilized to maintain differences across potentially excitable cell membranes, including the cardiac muscle. Intracellular calcium levels are relatively low compared to extracellular levels, and storage is within the mitochondria and organelles. Release of calcium from the intracellular space is carried out by transport of calcium out of the intracellular space by transport proteins. Calcium can also be removed from the intracellular space by hydrolysis of ATP to pump calcium out of the cell via the plasma membrane (Fleming 1980).

Voltage-dependent calcium selective channels are important for synaptic transmission through the release of neurotransmitters. Chemical synapses allow communication between the patient's non-neuronal cells and neuronal cells, allowing transmission of signals to the brain. Non-neuronal cells would commonly be described as those of muscle, soft tissue, and glands. The process begins with an "action potential" at the cell membrane, traveling until it reaches the synapse. There is then electrical depolarization, which allows calcium channels to open. Calcium ions flow into the intracellular space rapidly increasing the intracellular calcium levels and subsequently the amount of energy that particular cell can create for essential function. The role of calcium ions is diverse and at any one time there are various functions being carried out by calcium ions—from the stimulation of release of a hormone and triggering a muscle contraction to triggering neurotransmission. There are different types of calcium channels in the body and they will all behave in a slightly different way depending upon the role they carry out. As ions carry a small electrical charge, they can generate the energy to carry out these essential roles. Equally, if there is disruption of the number of calcium ions, the homeostatic mechanisms are not functioning, or there is damage at a cellular level, we will see disruption of calcium homeostasis and the detrimental effects that accompany that (Schenck et al. 1996; Rasmussen et al. 1990; Fleming 1980).

Accurate sampling techniques are important, and inappropriate handling, storage of blood before testing, or using certain anticoagulants can lead to sampling errors. If we are considering the biologically available calcium (ionized) then levels can be obtained both aerobically and anaerobically; however, the PH of the sample is important and the most precise determination of ionized calcium will come from a sample obtained and stored anaerobically to ensure no increase in PH. Ionized calcium and PH are most stable if there is a delay in analysis in serum samples (Larsson & Ohman 1985). Calcium measurements can be accurately monitored from serum or heparinized plasma. Calcium binds to certain chemicals and becomes unavailable for analysis. This would include oxalate, citrate, and EDTA as anticoagulants. Other factors which may affect calcium analysis (Table 7.1) include hemolysis, which falsely increases calcium levels; underfilled sampling tubes; lipemia, which can lead to false readings; and patients with increased levels of bilirubin, which can lead to decreased calcium levels on analysis (Larsson & Ohman 1985; Meuten 1984).

Table 7.1 Factors affecting calcium analysis when sampling

Anti-coagulant type	EDTA, oxalate and citrate will give erroneous results due to being calcium binding agents
Sample storage	Samples stored in a manner that allows changes in PH may give inaccurate readings
Sampling technique	Hemolysis will affect measurements due to destruction of cells
Under filling of sampling tubes	Results will be inaccurate
Other factors	Lipemia and hyperbilirubinemia can lead to inaccurate results

Hypocalcemia

Hypocalcemia in small animals can occur for multiple reasons. Any disease process affecting the intake, absorption, storage, or excretion of calcium may result in hypocalcemia. Alongside this, any disease affecting the calcium regulatory hormones or disorders of the homeostatic mechanisms involved can cause disorders resulting in hypocalcemia.

Hypocalcemia causes excitability of the peripheral and central nervous systems—this may be subclinical and in fact often is not seen. The severity of hypocalcemia is often dependent upon the duration and rate of decline of ionized calcium. Typical expected clinical signs in acute hypocalcemia include muscle tremors and twitches, and tetany can occur where compensatory mechanisms have failed (Petersen 2013a). Calcium creates energy for cells and if there is a reduction in the normal low level of calcium and cell membrane excitability the energy normally utilized for cellular function is depleted over a period of time in these patients. In the hypocalcemic patient, low levels of calcium increase the cell membrane excitability, leading to clinical signs such as tremors, twitching, and convulsions. Hypocalcemia, particularly in its acute and severe form, can lead to death due to decreased myocardial contractility and respiratory arrest due to paralysis of respiratory muscles as well as hypotension (Drop 1985; Feldman & Nelson 2004). Hypocalcemia will be present when there is either a decreased intake of dietary calcium over a period of time, a lack of regulatory hormone effect such as reduced or absent PTH excretion, problems with the production of vitamin D or calcitriol, and in patients where absolute body levels of calcium have been depleted and are not being replaced enterically. Central nervous system signs are similar to those of idiopathic epilepsy; however, if undiagnosed, seizure activity will be more frequent and resemble status epilepticus, including major convulsions with tonic-clonic seizure activity until calcium is supplemented (Dhupa & Proulx 1998; Sherding et al. 1980).

Hypocalcemia can be caused by underlying disease states, such as acute or chronic kidney disease, pancreatitis, sepsis, poor enteric absorption, and either an acquired or actual parathyroid disease process affecting PTH synthesis and production as well as storage, absorption, and excretion disorders. Many patients may have a subclinical hypocalcemia which is asymptomatic outwardly; however due to the requirement of calcium for cellular health, coagulation, and appropriate muscle contraction and energy production for the ATP pump, a subclinical hypocalcemia may require treatment depending upon the severity and if the reduction in ionized calcium is prolonged or transient. Due to calcium being required to provide energy for cellular function, we may see asymptomatic patients upon presentation; however, when we begin to address the underlying disease state and improve perfusion and oxygen delivery to the cells, they can become symptomatic. See Figure 7.2.

While chronic hypocalcemia is not in itself a diagnosis, it can be seen with various conditions in veterinary patients with varying severity. As patients may

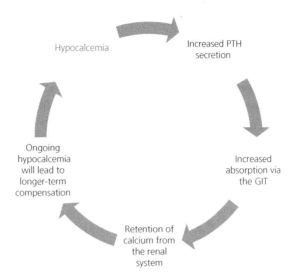

Figure 7.2 Initial response to hypocalcemia.

have multiple electrolyte disorders, changes in calcium levels may be present either at presentation, or develop as treatment for other disorders is performed. This is due to the relationship between calcium ions and other electrolyte ions at the cellular level, which can lead to the influx of ions through calcium channels, resulting in rapid changes of plasma calcium levels. Persistent hypocalcemia causes dysfunction of the neurons in the central nervous system, which affects musculoskeletal control and is why we can see twitching, tremors, and hyperexcitability (Drop 1985; Feldman & Nelson 2004).

For any patient that has reduced intake of calcium or vitamin D or ongoing consumption of calcium +/− elevated phosphorous or inappropriate calcium: phosphorous ratio has the potential to develop prolonged symptomatic hypocalcemia.

It is important to be aware that a patient can have normal total serum calcium but remain hypocalcemic—the most bioavailable source of calcium is ionized calcium. As such, calcium ions that are bound to proteins either in storage or buffering system or stored within the skeletal system are not readily available during an episode of hypocalcemia. In many patients the compensatory mechanisms including increased PTH secretion leading to increased enteric absorption will maintain normocalcemia. The issues we generally encounter in these patients occur because of ongoing utilization of the skeletally stored calcium with inappropriate replacement, poor absorption, or excessive excretion in the urine.

Eclampsia (puerperal tetany)

One of the most common acute severe presentations of hypocalcemia that will require emergency treatment we see in practice is the lactating bitch or queen. Although the presentation and development of clinical signs is often acute, the likelihood is the patient will have had a subclinical hypocalcemia for a period of time before displaying acute clinical signs.

Due to the increased metabolic demands of a nursing queen or bitch, they require a higher intake of calcium to maintain skeletal accumulation as well as the calcium required to be provided in the milk supply. In cases of eclampsia, patients often nurse large litters or are small patients with large neonates and their intake of calcium is insufficient to meet the demand for serum and milk calcium levels. There will be an increase in levels of PTH production, as described above, and a subsequent increase of absorption of calcium from the GIT as well as reabsorption from the renal system. There will also be mobilization of calcium from the ECF as well as calcitriol excretion to attempt to maintain calcium levels. This, however, can only compensate for a short period of time—if we recall that only a small amount of calcium is actually available to be mobilized from the skeletal system and it would be utilized rapidly in a patient that requires higher consumption over a prolonged period of time. These patients are likely to have a parathyroid independent hypocalcemia, as they will still be producing PTH—it is a matter of consumption of calcium ingested, absorbed, and stored within the body rather than an inability to synthesize PTH, vitamin D and calcitriol. With the effects of calcium at a cellular level causing excitability, we need to remember that this excitability can affect the cardiac muscle. We will normally see a rapid normalization of serum calcium levels with appropriate supplementation and reduction of clinical signs of hypocalcemia. However, this will only be effective long term if these patients are also given ongoing supplementation via dietary intake for the period of time that they have an increased calcium requirement (Sherding et al. 1980; Austad & Bjerkas 1976; Capen & Martin 1977; Care 1991).

Renal failure

Chronic renal failure can lead to hypocalcemia due to inefficient use of calcitonin. In chronic renal failure the kidney tubules, cells, and tissues will become damaged due to prolonged vasoconstriction leading to reduced glomerular filtration rates, which subsequently result in damage to the target cells that calcitonin works upon. Calcitonin is secreted from the C cells of the thyroid gland and targets receptors in the skeletal and renal system (Chew & Meuten 1982). In the presence of hypocalcemia in the ECF then calcitonin secretion will be increased initially. However, if there is damage to the target cells within the renal system that calcitonin would normally exert an effect upon, then the action of calcitonin will be suppressed and the normal response to hypocalcemia will become less efficient. Total serum calcium is often decreased in patients with chronic renal failure. However, these patients will often be asymptomatic due to increased ionized calcium that is normally associated with metabolic acidosis. Calcitriol deficits are more of a concern as hypocalcemia globally results from reduced intestinal absorption and increased skeletal resistance to PTH, meaning that absorption of calcium is reduced and the effects of PTH are ineffective due to calcitriol deficiency (Chew & Meuten 1982; Nagode & Chew 1991; Cortadellas et al. 2010).

Parathyroid hormone is perhaps characterized as a uremic toxin due to a combination of factors. These include mild hypocalcemia, reduction in the production of calcitriol, accumulation of phosphorous, and as the disease progresses a reduction in the number of vitamin D receptors (VDRs), meaning the effects that calcium in the ECF and calcitriol produced no longer exert control on the parathyroid glands. Hypocalcemia can play a major role in secondary renal hyperparathyroidism and bone demineralization (Rodriguez & Lorenzo 2009; Morrow & Volmer 2002).

There is also a recognized syndrome of chronic kidney disease mineral and bone disorder, which is characterized in the patient with chronic renal disease by uremic patients that have a high mineral and bone turnover. Increased levels of phosphorous compete with calcium for storage within the skeleton and lead to a condition whereby phosphorous is stored and calcium is excreted (Rodriguez & Lorenzo 2009; Morrow & Volmer 2002).

Hypoalbuminemia or conditions that lead to hypoproteinemia such as sepsis, malabsorption syndromes, and starvation may lead to a global hypocalcemia due to the buffering, storage, and transport systems associated with serum proteins. In these patients, hypocalcemia is normally mild and asymptomatic and should resolve with appropriate treatment for the underlying condition. As there is a large amount of total calcium bound to, stored, and buffered by proteins, hypoalbuminemia can cause a total hypocalcemia with a normal ionized calcium level. Even though the amount of calcium bound to proteins is significant, it may not be readily available in the face of hypocalcemia because proteins serve as storage and are used in buffering, but are not an active component of calcium homeostasis. Clinical signs of hypocalcemia are not normally seen in these patients (Ettinger & Feldman 2010; Chew & Meuten 1982).

Critically ill patients

In patients presented as emergency or critical care patients, there are likely to be multiple acid-base and electrolyte imbalances. Some may be due to the underlying disease process; others may be due to the primary problem. In patients presenting as an emergency, acid-base and electrolyte assessment is crucial and ongoing monitoring is often required. Hypocalcemia in patients with critical illness is well documented in human intensive care patients. Due to the many different body systems affected in critical illness in animals and the fact we can have multi-organ dysfunction as well as reduced intake and absorption of calcium and vitamin D from the gastrointestinal system, PTH synthesis and action, calcitriol and calcitonin secretion, and vitamin D metabolism can all be affected. Calcium binding to proteins can also be affected in critical illness due to many of these patients either presenting with or developing a hypoproteinemia at some stage during their treatment. In addition to this, many emergency and critical care patients will normally have a period of reduced calcium intake from their diet due to anorexia, and may be unable to efficiently absorb calcium enterically.

Many disease processes are considered to be associated with hypocalcemia, including sepsis, systemic inflammatory response syndrome, hypomagnesemia, and acute intrinsic renal failure, which is more common in critical patients than those with chronic renal disease (Dhupa & Proulx 1998; Carlstedt et al. 1998; Zaloga & Chernow 1987; Zivin et al. 2001).

Acute pancreatitis may be associated with hypocalcemia. In our patients, free fatty acids are bound to the albumin molecule alongside calcium and in pancreatitis patients or those with increased free fatty acid circulation. As a consequence of the seemingly higher levels of calcium bound to proteins, the ionized calcium levels fall. Suggested mechanisms of action for low ionized calcium in these patients could also include PTH resistance, increased calcitonin production in the presence of glucoganemia, as well as deposits of calcium into the peripancreatic fat. PTH resistance or a deficit of PTH may be a result of hypomagnesemia, and as such magnesium levels should be monitored in any emergency patient (Petersen 2013a).

Patients presenting following vehicular trauma may show a hypocalcemia due to muscle trauma or muscle necrosis. Alongside measurement of total and ionized calcium, it would be advisable in patients that have received any injury to the musculoskeletal system to monitor creatinine kinase levels as this is a specific indicator for muscular damage. Hypocalcemia in these patients likely occurs due to relocation of calcium into the muscle tissue. It is normally mild and not clinically relevant. Crush and traumatic injuries that cause damage to muscle cells or blood supply to the muscles or other non-physical injuries can interfere with cellular metabolism and production of energy. Damaged muscular cells will rapidly fill with fluid from the circulation, including an influx of sodium ions and cellular swelling. Damage to muscle cells can also lead to an influx of calcium and sodium ions across the calcium channels affecting the contractility of the cells and on occasion leading to continuous cellular contraction. If cells are contained in the muscles, muscle contraction may in turn deplete the energy used by the cell (ATP). When ATP (which is the primary currency of energy for many cells) is depleted, this can lead to further influx of calcium ions in an uncontrolled fashion into the intracellular space leading to cellular damage and death due to breakdown of intracellular proteins. When intracellular proteins breakdown, there is no mechanism for transport of calcium ions into and out of the cellular space (Dhupa & Proulx 1998; Gaschen et al. 1998).

Gastrointestinal disease may present patients with a mild hypocalcemia. Intake of calcium is dietary and as such relies upon a constant source of good-quality nutrition and appropriate absorption from the GIT alongside adequate vitamin D in the diet. Patients with gastrointestinal disease may have decreased intake or anorexia, leading to poor enteric absorption. Patients with damage to the villi and enterocytes lining the intestines, such as those with parvovirus, will have poor absorption of foods and transport of calcium and phosphate across the enterocytes leading to a dietary deficiency of calcium and vitamin D. Again, these patients commonly do not show clinical signs of hypocalcemia, and in many cases if the calcium regulatory hormone mechanisms remain functional, normocalcemia will resume once the GIT is healthy and the patient is receiving appropriate nutritional support.

Hypoparathyroidism is one of the major causes of severe symptomatic hypocalcemia and is normally present as a consequence of parathyroid hormone deficiency. With low or absent levels of PTH synthesis, patients are unable to metabolize and store calcium, leading to consumption of the calcium that can be mobilized from the skeletal system and eventually clinical signs of hypocalcemia. Hypocalcemia can be defined as parathyroid-dependent or parathyroid independent based upon the disease process.

The three main causes of hypoparathyroidism can be separated into three categories: (1) suppression of PTH secretion without damage or destruction to the parathyroid gland, (2) sudden correction of hypercalcemia, and (3) absence or destruction of the parathyroid gland (Dhupa & Proulx 1998; Chew & Meuten 1982; Schenck et al. 2012: 172–4).

The parathyroid gland is responsible for the major regulatory hormone associated with calcium storage and absorption, and as such any damage that leads to a reduction or cessation of PTH secretion can lead to hypocalcemia. It is uncommon for patients to develop primary hypoparathyroidism. However, it is possible if patients have the parathyroid gland removed—for example feline patients that have the parathyroid removed while thyroidectomy is being carried out or patients that have a parathyroid tumor. They will have a complete cessation of PTH production, and as such a hypocalcemia will follow due to no effects being exerted by PTH on absorption, storage, or mobilization of calcium (Dhupa & Proulx 1998; Birchard, Peterson, & Jacobson 1984; Flanders et al. 1987; Graves 1995).

There is the potential for idiopathic hypoparathyroidism in dogs. It is presumed to be caused by a diffuse lymphocytic inflammation of the parathyroid gland leading to damage of the chief cells within the gland and the cells becoming replaced with fibrous tissues. It is possible that there is an immune mediated component to this type of hypoparathyroidism. However, further investigation is required (Sherding et al. 1980).

Alongside the idiopathic or known causes of hypoparathyroidism (inadvertent removal of the parathyroid gland), the potential for tumors of the parathyroid gland and subsequent damage to the chief cells when associated with neoplasia can also be considered as important. Any disease process that damages the synthesis and secretion of PTH from the parathyroid gland will lead to hypocalcemia. It is also possible that the chief cells may lack the specific enzyme required to convert pro-PTH to PTH therefore making PTH biologically unavailable (Dhupa & Proulx 1998; Birchard, Peterson, & Jacobson 1984; Flanders et al. 1987; Graves 1995).

Hypercalcemia

Hypercalcemia is a less common clinical presentation. However, it is an important electrolyte disorder to consider, diagnose, and treat. High levels of calcium can affect cellular function and lead to dramatic and significant gastrointestinal, cardiovascular, neurologic, and renal dysfunction. The severity of the patient's clinical presentation will dictate how rapidly and aggressively these patients should be treated. Based upon the patients clinical presentation will dictate how rapidly and aggressively these patients require intervention. Due to the negative effects of high levels of calcium at a cellular level, we can see clinical signs of disease in any body system, though most commonly these will be evident in the body systems associated with calcium storage or excretion (Rasmussen et al. 1990; Rasmussen 1989).

The most common causes of hypercalcemia in small animal patients are malignant neoplasias, chronic renal failure, primary hyperparathyroidism, hypoadrenocorticism, hypervitaminosis D, and skeletal diseases associated with osteolysis and granulomatous inflammation. It should also be remembered that some patients at different life stages, such as growing patients, will have higher levels of calcium present, particularly ionized and in the ECF, depending on their requirement at different life stages (Petersen 2013b; Caldin et al. 2001).

The normal homeostatic response to correct hypercalcemia involves a reduction of the secretion of PTH, reducing the amount of calcium absorbed enterically and stored within the body. As well as suppression of PTH production, there will be an increase in degradation of PTH in the chief cells of the parathyroid gland leading to an overall reduction in the PTH availability to act upon calcium. Additionally, calcitonin release will be increased in an attempt to minimize the detrimental effects of hypercalcemia by increasing excretion via the renal system. In prolonged hypercalcemia, it is possible for the chief cells in parathyroid glands to become hyperplastic in an attempt to control calcium levels. Calcitriol levels are decreased in hypercalcemia through inhibition of ionized calcium alongside decreased stimulation due to a decrease in PTH secretion (Petersen 2013b; Caldin et al. 2001; Feldman & Nelson 2004; Box 7.1).

Hypocalcemia is normally an indicator of another disease process rather than a disease process in itself. It can be indicative of a disease state but can also cause

---

Box 7.1 Hypercalcemia and PTH

- PTH secretion is reduced, leading to reduced absorption from the GIT.
- Degradation of PTH in the parathyroid glands leads to less PTH being available to act upon calcium ions.
- Calcitonin production is increased, leading to increased renal excretion.
- Calcitriol levels are decreased following a decrease in PTH stimulation.

disease due to detrimental pathophysiologic damage. Therefore it is recommended that any patient with a consistent hypercalcemia should have investigations carried out to identify and treat the underlying issue (if there is one) or alternatively to attempt to reverse the detrimental effects high levels of calcium have at a tissue and cellular level. Calcium can be deposited into any tissue or organ and lead to mineralization or accumulation of calcium in the tissues leading to reduction of ATP production and ultimately cellular death as the ATP energy provision for cells becomes non-functional. Mineralization of the cardiac muscle and kidney is possible, leading to further complications due to distribution of excessive calcium into muscle and tissues (Rosol et al. 1995; Schenck, Chew, & Behrend 2006; Schenck et al. 2012: 134, 172–4).

Increase in either total or ionized serum calcium levels can lead to decreases in cellular function, due to alterations in cellular membrane permeability and decreased cellular energy production ultimately leading to cellular death. Changes in the exchange of sodium and potassium across the calcium channels and changes in the intracellular calcium levels are all cause for concern. The body systems affected by high calcium levels are multiple and should be considered. Skeletal muscle cells also suffer from the toxic effects of hypercalcemia and can manifest as patients showing signs of lethargy, weakness, and potentially mobility issues. Due to depression of cellular membrane excitability, we would not normally see seizure activity in hypercalcemic patients. However, we can see central nervous system signs due to cell toxicity. What we may see as central nervous system signs would include depression and lethargy due to the direct effects of hypercalcemia on the brain. We may also due to disruption of intracellular homeostasis, see an influx of sodium ions via the calcium channels leading to cellular swelling. These patients can occasionally develop cerebral edema, and sometimes, though rarely, these patients may become stuperous and comatose (Rosol et al. 1995; Bronner 2003; Chew & Meuten 1982; Rasmussen 1989).

Increased levels of serum or ionized calcium require certain mechanisms to be present which would include increases in calcium in the ECF, decreases in the amount of calcium utilized by the ECF, reduced plasma volumes which lead to hypercalcemia by hemoconcentration, or a combination of these factors. Additionally, increases in intestinal absorption, bone reabsorption, or renal reabsorption can lead to clinically significant hypercalcemia.

Hypercalcemia should be assessed as to the duration of the disease state, the severity of the hypercalcemia, and the way in which the patient is affected. Prolonged persistent hypercalcemic states are normally associated with a malignancy with the majority of studies in dogs attributing hypercalcemia to malignancy in around 50% of cases (Elliot et al. 1991).

In patients with mild or transient hypercalcemia, it can be more difficult to determine the cause, with occasional incidence of hypercalcemia accounting for hypoadrenocorticism, renal failure, primary hyperparathyroidism, hypervitaminosis D, and inflammatory disorders (Schenck et al. 2012: 134).

Renal failure

Hypercalcemia can occur in conjunction with chronic or acute intrinsic renal failure but high levels of calcium can also contribute to or worsen the disease process due to mineralization presenting within the renal tissue. Hypercalcemia can cause renal vasoconstriction leading to a reduced glomerular filtration rate and renal blood flow. Impaired renal function and renal autoregulation may result in azotemia in early stages of dehydration of a hypercalcemic patient. Acute intrinsic renal failure occasionally develops as a result of hypercalcemia; however, more commonly, chronic intrinsic renal failure will become worse due to sustained renal vasoconstriction, and may result in ischemic tubular injury. As we know that elevated calcium levels themselves can cause renal failure and we can also have elevated calcium as a result of renal failure, it can sometimes be difficult to differentiate between the cause and effect. Understanding that elevated levels of calcium can lead to tissue necrosis, cellular death, and renal vasoconstriction with reduced glomerular filtration rates is important when considering treatment options. Polydipsia and/or polyuria (PD/PU) may be seen as clinical signs of hypercalcemia. Hypercalcemia has a direct effect on the thirst center in the hypothalamus, which causes the patient to drink more and subsequently urinate more than usual, in an effort to excrete more calcium. If the effect of calcitonin is not efficient within the renal system, however, the patient's calcium levels will not fall and the phosphorous levels will rise. We can also see muscular weakness, ataxia, and dehydration. It should be noted that a patient with hypercalcemia and signs of azotemia, such as increased blood urea nitrogen and creatinine levels alongside an inability to concentrate urine, may not have developed renal failure, as all of these abnormalities can be due to an increased ionized calcium level as the primary cause (Schenck, Chew, & Behrend 2006; Galvao et al. 2013; Fleming 1980).

Patients with renal failure may develop secondary hyperparathyroidism due to calcitriol in the early disease stage diminishing parathyroid hormone synthesis. Calcitriol interacts with the vitamin D receptors in a wide variety of tissues throughout the body, and if a combination of phosphorous restriction which prevents tissue mineralization is used then calcitriol supplementation may also be beneficial to lower parathyroid hormone levels (Nagode, Chew, & Podell 1996). Long-term calcitriol deficits will lead to increased parathyroid hormone levels. However, with secondary hyperparathyroidism, the increases in parathyroid hormone and subsequent reduction in calcitriol production leads to the potential for widespread damage occurring in any tissue that has parathyroid receptors within the body (Hazewinkel 1991).

Hypercalcemia in cancer

Cancer is the most common cause of prolonged persistent hypercalcemia in dogs and the third most common cause of hypercalcemia in cats. Increases in calcium where there is either destruction of the bone from primary malignant bone cancers, such as osteosarcoma or metastases from a primary site are often seen. This is caused

Table 7.2 Common cancers and incidence of hypercalcemia

Type of cancer	Incidence of hypercalcemia
Lymphosarcoma	20–40%
Adenocarcinoma	80–100%
Multiple myeloma	17%

by systemically acting humoral factors released by the neoplasia and affecting the absorption and excretion of calcium at the receptors in the intestine, bone, and kidneys. In these patients the hypercalcemia would be classed as parathyroid independent as there should still be secretion of calcium regulatory hormones. There are three mechanisms of induced hypercalcemia in neoplastic disease which include (1) humoral hypercalcemia of malignancy, (2) local osteolytic hypercalcemia occurs when there are metastases of solid tumors, and (3) malignancies of the bone marrow (hematological) (Rosol & Capen 1992, 2000).

Humoral hypercalcemia of malignancy is characterized by hypercalcemia in the presence of a neoplastic or malignant process. We will commonly encounter hypophosphatemia, increases in excretion of phosphorus, and increased osteoclastic bone resorption. Osteoclast-activating factors in these cases are released far from the malignant cells, leading to an increase in bone resorption and a subsequent increase in calcium from the bone, alongside inappropriate exchange of calcium and phosphorous out of the skeletal system and into the bloodstream. In the pathogenesis of hypercalcemia, the kidney plays a vital role in the development of hypercalcemia and the level of renal function the patient has becomes important. Any patient with impaired renal function, dehydration, or reduced glomerular filtration rates may be more at risk from hypercalcemia due to poor calcium excretion via the kidneys alongside hyperphosphatemia. There is a specific protein for parathyroid hormone (PTHrP), and excessive secretion of this in a biologically active state can play a major role in humoral hypercalcemia of malignancy. However, there will be other factors to consider, including cytokines, tumor necrosis factors, and transforming growth factors. Calcitriol may work synergistically with PTHrP. PTHrP increases intracellular calcium in the skeletal and renal systems through a process of binding to cell membranes and activation. This stimulates osteoclastic bone resorption as well as increases renal tubule calcium resorption and decreases renal phosphate absorption (Rosol & Capen 1988, 1992, 2000). The most common types of cancer seen in small animal patients causing a subsequent hypercalcemia are shown in Table 7.2.

Lymphoma

Most patients presenting with hypercalcemia and lymphoma will have a humoral hypercalcemia of malignancy and will usually be associated with T-cell lymphoma (Rosol & Capen 1992). Lymphocytes in some cases retain the ability to convert vitamin D to the active metabolite of calcitriol, and as such this may lead to increased absorption of calcium from the GIT. Hypercalcemia is associated with increased osteoclastic bone resorption without evidence of metastasis.

Adenocarcinoma

Many of these patients will be presented with clinical signs of hypercalcemia including polydipsia, polyuria, anorexia, and weakness associated with cellular toxicity arising from increased levels of calcium. These patients consistently fulfill the criteria of humoral hypercalcemia of malignancy without metastases to the bone (Rosol & Capen 1988, 1992, 2000; Meuten et al. 1983). Adenocarcinomas derived from the apocrine glands of the anal sacs should not be confused with perianal adenomas, which act differently. Adenocarcinomas have a wide range of size from 7 mm to 6 × 8 cm. These patients will commonly, alongside the hypercalcemia, have an increase in urinary excretion of calcium and phosphorous as well as increased osteoclastic bone resorption (Rosol & Capen 1992, 1998, 2000; Meuten et al. 1983). Hypercalcemia has not been confirmed as a prognostic indicator in these patients, with one study suggesting these patients would survive longer if they had normocalcemia at the time of presentation and another showing no correlation (Meuten et al. 1983; Bennett et al. 2000; Williams et al. 2003). Many patients with apocrine adenocarcinomas were found to have atrophied or non-functional parathyroid glands due to prolonged hypercalcemia. We may also see increased plasma PTHrP concentrations in these patients, which would confirm the activity of PTHrP and its pathogenesis in patients with humoral hypercalcemia of malignancy (Rosol et al. 1992).

Hematological malignancies

These are commonly considered as cancers that present in the bone marrow and cause local bone resorption (Rosol & Capen 1988, 1992, 2000). These patients will often have a hypercalcemia with a reduction in PTH and calcitriol concentrations and increased secretion of calcium and phosphorous. Hypercalcemia is most commonly seen in patients with lymphoma or multiple myeloma, and there are a number of factors which may lead to development of hypercalcemia in these patients, including production of small amounts of PTHrP from the tumors themselves that can stimulate local resorption of bone (Williams et al. 2003).

Tumors metastatic to bone

Some solid tumors that metastasize widely to the bone can cause hypercalcemia due to increases in local bone resorption. This is a common cause of malignancy-induced hypercalcemia in humans (Rosol & Capen 2000; Rosol et al. 2004). In small animal patients it is uncommon. Enhanced bone resorption in malignancy is likely caused by two primary mechanisms, including secretion of cytokines that stimulate local bone resorption and cytokine secretion from local immune or bone cells (Rosol et al. 2004).

Whilst there are other causes for hypercalcemia the most common recognized cause is normally a malignancy in patients that have ongoing, persistent hypercalcemia. When we consider cancers of malignancy it is important to understand the characteristic findings associated with this. We will often find these patients have hypercalcemia, hypophosphatemia, and increased osteoclastic bone resorption. Tumors that metastasize widely to the bone produce hypercalcemia associated with the rate of growth of the tumor (Rosol & Capen 1988, 1992; Meuten et al. 1983; Williams et al. 2003; Rosol et al. 1992).

Hypervitaminosis D

Hypervitaminosis D is normally a result of intoxication resulting from the major vitamin D metabolites, either cholecalciferol (D3) or ergocalciferol (D2), although the majority of metabolites of vitamin D are capable of causing toxicity. Hypercalcemic effects are seen when there is competition at the vitamin D receptors in target tissues against calcitriol. There is a subsequent increase in intestinal reabsorption of calcium. There are several causes of vitamin D intoxication, due to the slow onset of action. When vitamin D is given as a treatment option, we can also induce a hypervitaminosis D in patients undergoing treatment for hypoparathyroidism (Chew & Meuten 1982; Schenck et al. 2012: 155). Other causes include excessive dietary intake or supplementation. With there being no guidance for commercial food companies as to how much is the upper limit of vitamin D allowed in foods, some commercial foods have been recorded as having up to 100 times the recommended daily amount (Freeman et al. 2013).

There is also the potential for patients to ingest cholecalciferol by eating certain plants, namely *Cestrum diurnum* (day-blooming jessamine), which has grown in popularity as a house plant and has active vitamin D metabolites (Drazner 1981). Cholecalciferol is also contained within some rodenticides and this should be explored as a possible cause of toxicity in the event of hypervitaminosis D being diagnosed for an unknown cause. Alongside the deleterious effects of hypercalcemia, we can also see disorders in coagulation as the elevated calcium levels will disrupt the coagulation cascade. Hypercalcemia in these cases is often severe within 24 hr of ingestion and requires aggressive therapy to reverse the toxicity. The dangers of cholecalciferol particularly are its extremely long half-life which can subsequently lead to ongoing prolonged toxic effects (Schenck et al. 2012: 155; Drazner 1981). Serum calcitriol levels are elevated early in the syndrome; however, as they continue to compete with the vitamin D metabolites, azotemia develops and suppression of calcitriol synthesis occurs.

Idiopathic hypercalcemia in cats

Hypercalcemia with no recognizable clinical cause has become more common in the United States feline population over the last 15–20 years. Prolonged hypercalcemia has been recognized in some feline patients with no known cause despite extensive investigations. There have been some suggestions that there is a geographical connection with these patients. However, this has not been proven and cases of idiopathic hypercalcemia are being recorded in other areas. Serum calcium concentrations in these patients may be elevated for months with no clinical signs, or non-specific signs such as gastrointestinal disorders. On occasion these patients will have uroliths or renoliths, and calcium oxalate stones have been noted in some cases (Schenck et al. 2004).

The pathogenesis of this disease remains unknown with PTH concentration remaining normal, vitamin D levels within the normal range, and mild suppression of calcitriol as would be expected in a hypercalcemic patient. Any combination of mechanisms could be responsible for this idiopathic disorder, including increased dietary intake, bone resorption, or intestinal absorption, with or without decreased renal excretion.

Hyperparathyroidism

Primary hyperparathyroidism may occur in dogs and cats but is an uncommon cause of hypercalcemia. In this condition the parathyroid gland excretes parathyroid hormone at excessive levels in relation to the serum ionized calcium levels. In approximately 90% of cases in the canine population the cause of hypoparathyroidism was a parathyroid gland adenoma. The mechanism of disease for patients with hyperparathyroidism is thought to be a combination of effects.

- Parathyroid hormone is secreted at levels that are inappropriate to the ionized calcium concentration, leading to increased bone resorption allowing release of calcium from the skeletal system to the circulating blood volume. PTH also indirectly increases ionized calcium concentration by increasing vitamin D conversion to calcitriol.
- Serum levels of phosphorous are typically low due to increased excretion via the kidneys.
- Increased intestinal calcium absorption occurs in response to the elevated PTH levels.

Treatment of hypercalcemia associated with hyperparathyroidism will rely upon identification of the underlying cause and treatment where possible. Parathyroid gland tumors can potentially be removed or treated using ultrasonically guided radiofrequency heat ablation. These patients should have their ionized and total calcium levels monitored closely as they will potentially develop hypocalcemia (Schenck et al. 2012: 134; Elliot et al. 1991; Rosol & Capen 2000).

Treatment of hypercalcemia generally relies on identification of the underlying cause. Supportive therapies may include intravenous fluid therapy, the use of loop diuretics such as furosemide to increase excretion, inhibiting absorption of calcium across the GIT, and causing a shift of calcium into the body compartments. There are, of course, other treatment options and considerations for the hypercalcemic patient, and these will need to be assessed on a case-by-case basis dependent on the duration of the disease process and the potential for the hypercalcemia to have caused damage in tissues and cells.

It would be expected to be normal to have some variation in calcium levels dependent upon the patient's life stage, dietary intake of calcium, and other day-by-day changes in homeostasis. It is important to recognize the different factors affecting calcium regulation and the potential for inappropriate calcium levels causing severe disruption in body systems.

References

Austad, R. & Bjerkas, E. (1976). Eclampsia in the bitch. *Journal of Small Animal Practice* **17**: 793–8.

Barrette, D. C. (1988). Calcium and phosphorus for cats and dogs. *Canadian Veterinary Journal* **29**(9): 751.

Bennett, P. F., DeNicola, D. B., Bonney, P., et al. (2000). Canine anal sac adenocarcinomas: Clinical presentation and response to therapy. *Journal of Veterinary Internal Medicine* **16**: 100–104.

Birchard, S. J., Peterson, M. E., & Jacobson, A. (1984). Surgical treatment of feline hyperthyroidism: Results of 85 cases. *Journal of the American Animal Hospital Association* **20**:705–9.

Bowen, R. (2011). Vitamin D (calcitriol), http://www.vivo.colostate.edu/hbooks/pathphys/endocrine/otherendo/vitamind.html.

Bronner, F. (2003). Mechanisms of intestinal calcium absorption. *Journal of Cellular Biochemistry* **88**: 387–93.

Caldin, M., Tomasso, F., Lubas, G. et al. (2001). Incidence of persistent hypercalcemia in dogs and its diagnostic approach. *European Society of Veterinary Internal Medicine Congress*, Dublin, Ireland.

Capen, C. C. & Martin, S. L. (1977). Calcium metabolism and disorders of parathyroid glands. *Veterinary Clinics of North America* **7**: 513–548.

Care, A. D. (1991). The placental transfer of calcium. *Journal of Developmental Physiology* **15**: 253–7.

Carlstedt, F., Lind, L., Rastad, J., et al. (1998). Parathyroid hormone and ionized calcium levels related to the severity of illness and survival in critically ill patients. *European Journal of Clinical Investigation* **28**: 898–903.

Chew, D. J. & Meuten, D. J. (1982). Disorders of calcium and phosphorous metabolism. *Veterinary Clinics of North America: Small animal practice* **12**: 411–438.

Cortadellas, O., Fernandez del Palacio, M. J., Talavera, J., & Bayón, A. (2010). Calcium and phosphorus homeostasis in dogs with spontaneous chronic kidney disease at different stages of severity. *Journal of Veterinary Internal Medicine* **24**(1): 73–9.

Deluca, H. F., Krisinger, J., & Darwish, H. (1990). The Vitamin D system. *Kidney International Supplements* **29**: S2–8.

Dhupa, N. & Proulx, J. (1998). Hypocalcaemia and hypomagnesia. *Veterinary Clinics of North America: Small animal practice* **28**: 586–608.

DiBartola, S. P. (ed.), (2012). Disorders of calcium. In: *Fluid, Electrolyte, and Acid-Base Disorders in Small Animal Practice*, 4th ed. St Louis, MO: W. B. Saunders: 126–8.

Drazner, F. H. (1981). Hypercalcemia in the dog and cat. *Journal of the American Veterinary Medical Association* **178**: 1252–6.

Drop, L. J. (1985). Ionized calcium and, the heart and haemodynamic function. *Anesthesia & Analgesia* **64**: 432–51.

Elliot, J., Dobson, J., Dunn, J. et al. (1991). Hypercalceamia in the dog. *Journal of Small Animal Practice* **32**: 564–71.

Ettinger, S. J. & Feldman, E. C. (2010). *Textbook of Veterinary Internal Medicine*. St Louis, MO: Saunders.

Feldman, E. C. & Nelson, R. W. (2004). Hypocalcemia and primary hypoparathyrodism. In: E. C. Feldman (ed.), *Canine and Feline Endocrinology and Reproduction*. St Louis, MO: W. B. Saunders: 660–715.

Flanders, J. A., Harvey, H. J., Erb, H. N., et al. (1987). Feline thyroidectomy: A comparison of postoperative hypocalcaemia associated with three different surgical techniques. *Veterinary Surgery* **16**: 362–6.

Fleming, W. W. (1980). The electrogenic Na$^+$, K$^+$ pump in smooth muscle: Physiologic and pharmacologic significance. *Annual Review of Pharmacology and Toxicology* **20**: 129–49.

Freeman, L. M., Chandler, M. L., Hamper, B. A., & Weeth, L. P. et al. (2013). Current knowledge about the risks and benefits of raw meat–based diets for dogs and cats. *JAVMA* **243**(11).

Galvao, J. F. B., Nagode, L., Schenck, P., & Chew, D. J. (2013). Calcitriol, calcidiol, parathyroid hormone and fibroblast growth factor-23 interactions in chronic kidney disease. *Journal of Veterinary Emergency & Critical Care* **23**(2): 134–62.

Gaschen, F., Gaschen, L., Seiler, G. et al. (1998). Lethal peracute rhabdomyolysis associated with stress and general anaesthesia in three dystrophin deficient cats. *Veterinary Pathology* **35**:117–123.

Graves, T. K. (1995). Complications of treatment and concurrent illness associated with hyperthyroidism in cats. In: J. D. Bonagura (ed.), *Kirk's Current Veterinary Therapy XII: Small animal practice*. St Louis, MO: W. B. Saunders: 369–72.

Hazewinkel, H. A. (1991). Dietary influences on calcium homeostasis and the skeleton. *Proceedings of the Purina International Nutrition Symposium, Eastern States Veterinary Conference*: 51–9.

Kronenberg, H. M., Bringhurst, F. R., Segre, G. V. et al. (2001). Parathyroid hormone biosynthesis and metabolism. In: J. P. Bilezikian, R. Marcus, & M. A. Levine (eds), *The Parathyroids*, 2nd ed. San Diego: Academic Press: 293–329.

Larsson, L., Ohman, S. (1985). Effect of silicone-separator tubes and storage time on ionized calcium in serum. *Clinical Chemistry* **31**: 169–70.

Massry, S. G. & Glassock, R. J. (2001). *Massry & Glassock's Textbook of Nephrology*. Philadelphia: Lippincott Williams & Wilkins.

Meuten, D. J. (1984). Hypercalcaemia. *Veterinary Clinics of North America* **14**: 891–910.

Meuten, D. J., Segre, G. V., Capen, C. C., et al. (1983). Hypercalcaemia associated with adenocarcinoma derived from the apocrine glands of the anal sac. Biochemical and histomorphometric investigations. *Laboratory Investigation* **48**: 428–35.

Morrow, C. K. & Volmer, P. A. (2002). Hypercalcemia, hyperphosphatemia, and soft-tissue mineralization. *Compendium* **24**(5): 380–388.

Nagode, L. A. & Chew, D. J. (1991). The use of calcitriol in treatment of renal disease of the dog and cat. *Proceedings of the 1st Purina International Nutrition Symposium*.

Nagode, L. A., Chew, D. J., & Podell, M. (1996). Benefits of calcitriol therapy and serum phosphorous control in dogs and cats with chronic renal failure. *Veterinary Clinics of North America: Small animal practice* **26**: 1293–1300.

Nagode, L. A., Chew, D. J., Steinmeyer, C. L. (1992). The use of low doses of calcitriol in the treatment of renal secondary hyperparathyroidism. *Proceedings of the 15th Waltham Symposium*.

Patel, S. R. Ke, H. Q., Vanholder, R. et al. (1995). Inhibition of calcitriol receptor binding to vitamin D response elements by ureamic toxins. *Journal of Clinical Investigation* **96**: 50–59.

Petersen, M. E. (2013a). Hypocalcemia in dogs and cats, http://www.merckmanuals.com/vet/endocrine_system/the_parathyroid_glands_and_disorders_of_calcium_metabolism/hypocalcemia_in_dogs_and_cats.html.

Petersen, M. E. (2013b). Hypercalcemia in dogs and cats, http://www.merckmanuals.com/vet/endocrine_system/the_parathyroid_glands_and_disorders_of_calcium_metabolism/hypercalcemia_in_dogs_and_cats.html.

Rasmussen, H. (1989). The cycling of calcium as an intracellular messenger. *Scientific American* **261**: 66–73.

Rasmussen, H., Barrett, P., Smallwood, J., et al. (1990). Calcium ion as intracellular messenger and cellular toxin. *Environmental Health Perspectives* **84**: 17–25.

Rodriguez, M. & Lorenzo, V. (2009). Parathyroid hormone: A ureamic toxin. *Seminars in Dialysis* **22**(4): 363–8.

Rosol, T. J. & Capen, C. C. (1988). Pathogenesis of humoral hypercalcaemia of malignancy. *Domestic Animal Endocrinology* **5**: 1–21.

Rosol, T. J. & Capen, C. C. (1992). Mechanisms of cancer induced hypercalcaemia *Laboratory Investigation* **67**: 680–702.

Rosol, T. J. & Capen, C. C. (2000). Cancer associated hypercalcaemia. In: B. F. Feldman, J. G. Zinkl, & N. C. Jain (eds), *Schalm's Veterinary Haematology* Philadelphia: Lippincott Williams & Wilkins: 600–666.

Rosol, T. J., Chew, D. J., Nagode, L. A., et al. (1995). Pathophysiology of calcium metabolism. *Veterinary Clinic Pathology* **24**: 49–63.

Rosol, T. J., Nagode, L. A., Couto, C. G., et al. (1992). Parathyroid hormone (PTH) related protein, PTH, and 1,25-dihydroxyvitamin D in dogs with cancer associated hypercalcaemia. *Endocrinology* **131**: 1157–64.

Rosol, T. J., Gregg, S. H., Corn, S., et al. (2004). Animal models of bone metastasis. *Cancer Treatment and Research* **118**: 47–81.

Schenck, P. A. & Chew, D. J. (2005). Prediction of serum ionized calcium concentration by use of serum total calcium concentration in dogs. *American Journal of Veterinary Research* **66**(8): 1330–1336.

Schenck, P. A., Chew, D. J., & Behrend, E. N. (2006). Updates on hypercalcemic disorders. In: J. R. August (ed.), *Consultations in Feline Internal Medicine*, 5th ed. St Louis, MO: W. B. Saunders: 157–68.

Schenck, P. A., Chew, D. J., & Brooks, C. L. (1996). Fractionation of canine serum calcium using a micropartition system. *American Journal of Veterinary Research* **57**: 268–71.

Schenck, P. A., Chew, D. J., Refsal, K., et al. (2004). Calcium metabolic hormones in feline idiopathic hypercalcaemia. *Journal of Veterinary Internal Medicine* **18**: 442.

Schenck, P., Chew, D. J., Nagode, L. A., & Rosol, T. J. (2012). Disorders of calcium: Hypercalceamia and hypocalcaemia. In: S. P. DiBartola (ed.), *Fluid, Electrolyte, and Acid-Base Disorders in Small Animal Practice*, 4th ed. St Louis, MO: W. B. Saunders.

Sherding, R. G., Meuten, D. J., Chew, D. J. et al. (1980). Primary hypoparathyroidism in the dog. *Journal of the American Veterinary Medical Association* **176**: 439–44.

Wasserman, R. H. (1981). Intestinal absorption of calcium and phosphorus. *Federation Proceedings* **40**(1): 68–72.

Williams, L. E., Gliattoo, J. M., Dodge, R. K., et al. (2003). Carcinoma of the apocrine glands of the anal sac in dogs: 113 cases 1985–1995. *Journal of the American Veterinary Medical Association* **223**: 825–31.

Zaloga, G. P. & Chernow, B. (1987). The multifactorial basis for hypocalcaemia during sepsis: Studies of the parathyroid hormone–Vitamin D axis. *Annals of Internal Medicine* **107**: 36–41.

Zivin, J. R., Gooley, T., Zager, R. A. et al. (2001). Hypocalcaemia: A pervasive metabolic abnormality in the critically ill. *American Journal of Kidney Diseases* **37**: 689–98.

CHAPTER 8

Traditional Acid-Base Physiology and Approach to Blood Gas

Jo Woodison, RVT and Angela Randels-Thorp, CVT, VTS (ECC, SAIM)

Introduction

The maintenance of a stable acid-base balance is a vital component of the body's homeostasis. Despite its importance, it is often a difficult or confusing mechanism to comprehend. In an effort to simplify the components that manage acid-base balance utilizing the traditional, or Henderson-Hasselbalch, approach can be broken down into two main systems: respiratory and metabolic.

The respiratory system is responsible for breathing, which is responsible for gas exchange in the lungs. When breathing is inadequate, carbon dioxide (CO_2, a respiratory acid) accumulates in the body, contributing to an acid state.

The metabolic system is responsible for a variety of chemical reactions that take place within a body's cells to convert the fuel supplied (food) into the energy used to power the body's functions, from basic operation at rest, to thinking, growing, and running, etc. When normal metabolism is impaired, acid will form. For example, when poor blood supply prevents aerobic metabolism, lactic acid forms, also contributing to an acid state.

The body's regulators of acid-base balance are primarily the lungs and the kidneys. In addition to contributing to an imbalance as just described, each system is able to compensate for a disturbance by secreting or retaining acid. When functioning correctly, the lungs can quite rapidly expel large quantities of carbon dioxide to reduce the quantity of acid in an effort to restore balance. The kidneys are slower to respond, but can also excrete more acid in their waste products, and retain more bicarbonate (HCO_3^-, a base or alkaline chemical), which is an important buffer employed within the body to help resolve or compensate for increased acid accumulation. In the cases where the body is too alkaline, or alkalosis has occurred, the respiratory system may become somewhat depressed to retain carbon dioxide; here the kidneys will play the more

Acid-Base and Electrolyte Handbook for Veterinary Technicians, First Edition.
Edited by Angela Randels-Thorp and David Liss.
© 2017 John Wiley & Sons, Inc. Published 2017 by John Wiley & Sons, Inc.
Companion website: www.wiley.com/go/liss/electrolytes

significant role and attempt to retain more acid and eliminate more bicarbonate (base substance) in an effort to maintain balance.

The majority of acid-base disturbances are classified into one of four types:

- Respiratory acidosis occurs when the lungs do not expel CO_2 adequately. There is an increase in CO_2, accompanied by a compensatory increase in HCO_3^-.
- Respiratory alkalosis occurs when too much CO_2 is expelled from the bloodstream (typically from hyperventilation). There is a decrease in CO_2 with a compensatory decrease in HCO_3^-.
- Metabolic acidosis occurs when there is an increase in the amount of acid in the body. This can be due to abnormal metabolic function, or ingestion of an acid or substance that is metabolized into an acid. There is a decrease in HCO_3^- and a compensatory decrease in CO_2.
- Metabolic alkalosis occurs when an excessive loss of sodium or potassium affects the kidney's ability to control the blood's acid-base balance. There is an increase in HCO_3^- and compensatory increase in CO_2.

Acid-base disorders frequently accompany critical illnesses. While they can be life-threatening themselves, they are usually secondary to another disease or ailment, such as sepsis, acute kidney injury, hemorrhage, trauma, severe metabolic dysregulation (e.g. diabetic ketoacidosis), and different types of shock.

Overview of acid-base

Key contributors to our understanding of blood gases and acid-base balance could be said to date back to the 1600s with Boyle's law, which (put very simply) states that pressure is inversely proportional to volume. There have been many discoveries between then and now and they are ongoing. The key developments in helping us understand how to approximate the pH of a buffer solution came from two scientists, who developed what is referred to as the Henderson–Hasselbalch equation. The contributors were Lawrence Joseph Henderson, a biochemist working at Harvard, who in 1908 discovered the buffering power of carbon dioxide and applied the law of mass action to it. His work was modified in 1916, by Karl Albert Hasselbalch, a chemist who studied pH closely. He also studied blood and the reactions that took place with oxygen. He modified Henderson's equation by adding mathematical logarithms to it, creating an improved relationship (Po & Shenozan 2001).

In the early 1980s, Peter A. Stewart, a Canadian physiologist, published a book (Stewart 1981) and then a paper (Stewart 1983) describing his concept of employing strong ion difference as an alternative means of assessing clinical acid-base disturbances. While interesting, even compelling, his work was not without criticism, and for most acid-base disturbances the traditional approach to acid-base balance has prevailed and will be discussed in this chapter. More detailed information pertaining to the Strong Ion approach to blood gas and acid-base measurement can be found in Chapter 12.

Acid-base balance refers to the physiologic mechanisms that the body employs to maintain the blood pH within the narrow range of 7.35–7.45. Recall that pH is a measure of the hydrogen ion (H^+, or "proton") concentration. More specifically, pH equals the inverse logarithm of the proton concentration.

$$pH = -\log[H^+]$$

As the number of protons increases, the pH decreases. A blood pH of less than 7.35 is termed acidemia, and a pH greater than 7.45 is known as alkalemia. Processes that tend to lower the pH are referred to as acidosis, and those that raise the pH are termed alkalosis.

Water (H_2O) and carbon dioxide (CO_2) are the primary substances in the body that determine acid-base balance. When present together, water and carbon dioxide combine to produce carbonic acid (H_2CO_3) in a reaction that is catalyzed by the enzyme carbonic anhydrase.

$$CO_2 + H_2O \longleftrightarrow H_2CO_3$$

Carbon dioxide is produced as a result of cellular respiration, and this can occur within any cell in the body. The majority is produced by the metabolism of carbohydrates and fats, with a much smaller quantity of non-volatile acid produced through protein metabolism. The lungs, liver, and kidneys jointly regulate the body's acid-base balance by controlling excretion and metabolism of these volatile and non-volatile acids. There are three primary mechanisms that control pH within the body to correct imbalances. Chemical buffers combine with acids or bases to prevent extreme changes in H^+ concentration, the respiratory center regulates the removal of CO_2 from the extracellular fluid (ECF), and the kidneys excrete either acidic or alkaline urine to help adjust ECF H^+ concentration.

Although carbon dioxide is not itself an acid, it readily combines with water to produce carbonic acid, and so it is often considered an acid in discussions of the body's acid-base balance. If carbon dioxide is not adequately exchanged with oxygen through alveolar respiration and excreted, acid quickly accumulates within the body. Given the ease and speed of carbonic acid formation from carbon dioxide, we can generally say that the greater the dissolved carbon dioxide concentration in the blood, the higher the carbonic acid concentration.

Bicarbonate (HCO_3^-) is another important molecule in the body's acid-base balance. The ratio of bicarbonate to carbon dioxide dictates the H^+ concentration, which is used in calculating pH. Our earlier equation can be expanded to show that carbon dioxide and water combine to produce carbonic acid, which in turn can be broken down into bicarbonate and H^+. The reverse reaction also occurs.

$$CO_2 + H_2O \longleftrightarrow H_2CO_3 \longleftrightarrow HCO_3^- + H^+$$

This equation describes the body's carbon dioxide–bicarbonate buffering system. The products on either side of this equation must balance; if one of the substances on the left increases, so must a substance on the right.

Buffer systems

Buffers are the first line of defense against acute changes in H⁺ concentration, or pH. A buffer is any compound that can either accepts or donates protons. Changes in pH are minimized because the buffer will accept protons (such as H⁺) when they are present in excess, and release ("donate") protons when there is a shortage. The body has several buffer systems within its extracellular (intravascular and interstitial) and intracellular compartments. The main buffering systems are:
- bicarbonate in plasma, interstitial and intracellular water, and carbonate in bone;
- intracellular proteins, including hemoglobin in red blood cells (RBCs);
- plasma proteins;
- intracellular and extracellular phosphates.

The extent to which buffer contributes to maintaining acid-base balance depends on the nature of the acid-base disturbance. Table 8.1 shows percentages of buffering provided by each buffer type.

Body buffers are generally weak acids. They readily dissociate and are able to accept or release protons, thereby minimizing changes to the overall free proton concentration, or pH. Bicarbonate is the most significant buffer in the ECF, and is present in appreciable quantities in nearly all body fluids. As described above, this buffer system consists of HCO_3^- combining with excess H⁺ to form H_2CO_3, which then dissociates into CO_2 and H_2O. The uncatalyzed reaction is slow, and

Table 8.1 Percentages of buffering provided by each buffer type (Source: Based on data from Hess, 2012)

Buffer type	% total buffering
Bicarbonate	**53**
• Plasma bicarbonate	35
• Erythrocyte bicarbonate	18
Non-bicarbonate	**47**
• Hemoglobin	35
• Organic phosphates	3
• Inorganic phosphates	2
• Plasma proteins	7
Total	**100**

only small amounts of H_2CO_3 are formed unless carbonic anhydrase is present to speed the reaction. This enzyme is abundant in the walls of the alveoli where CO_2 is released, and in the epithelial cells of the renal tubules where CO_2 reacts with H_2O to form H_2CO_3.

The lungs eliminate CO_2, while H_2O is excreted by the kidneys. Due to the ease of carbonic acid formation and subsequent dissociation, and because CO_2 can be eliminated rapidly by ventilation, H_2CO_3 is referred to as a volatile acid. Other metabolic acids, such as lactic acid, phosphoric acid, sulfuric acid, acetoacetic acid, and beta-hydroxybutyric acid, are referred to as fixed, or non-volatile, acids because they cannot be eliminated by the lungs. H^+ from these non-volatile acids can only be eliminated through the kidneys.

Because HCO_3^- is "used up" in the buffering reaction, it must be regenerated to maintain the body's primary buffer system and continued prevention of pH changes. The CO_2/HCO_3^- buffer system is effective and efficient due to the vast quantity of HCO_3^- present in the body, and the body's ability to quickly excrete the waste product CO_2 via ventilation. Other less significant buffers in the ECF include plasma proteins and inorganic phosphates.

Intracellular buffers include proteins, organic and inorganic phosphates, and hemoglobin (Hb^-). Hb^- is a very important buffer in RBCs, particularly with regards to the buffering of H_2CO_3. It is responsible for more than 80% of the non-bicarbonate buffering capacity. Plasma proteins, primarily albumin, make up the remaining 20%.

The CO_2/HCO_3^- buffer system is the system evaluated by arterial blood gas (ABG) analysis in clinical practice. [H^+] fluctuates based on changes in the ratio of HCO_3^- to carbonic acid (or CO_2). This relationship is described by the Henderson–Hasselbalch equation:

$$pH = 6.1 + \log\left[HCO_3^- / pCO_2 \times 0.03\right]$$

The number 6.1 is used in this equation because it is the logarithmic disassociation constant (pK_a) of carbonic acid (DiBartola 2012). The disassociation constant (K_a) measures the strength of an acid. Essentially, 6.1 represents the level of carbonic acid's tendency to break down into bicarbonate ions (HCO_3^-) and hydrogen ions (H^+). We do not generally measure carbonic acid in the blood but know that it readily converts to CO_2. Most laboratories and in-house analyzers do not measure actual CO_2 dissolved in blood, but the partial pressure of CO_2 in the blood (pCO_2). In calculating pH we multiply the pCO_2 by 0.03, (the solubility constant for CO_2 in plasma) (Rose 2001) to approximate the carbonic acid concentration. This signifies that at a normal body temperature, 0.03 mmol of H_2CO_3 is present in the blood for every 1 mmHg pCO_2 measured.

Acid-base disturbances

Acid-base disturbances are the result of an imbalance between the quantity of acids produced and the body's ability to respond and neutralize these acids. The most common scenario seen in clinical practice is a characteristic, partial compensation for any imbalance.

Remember that pH is an inverse logarithm of the proton concentration: an increase in H^+ concentration causes a reduction in blood pH (acidemia), and a decrease in H^+ concentration causes an increase in pH (alkalemia). Management of CO_2 levels within the body is handled by the brain's respiratory center, working together with the lungs, and resulting changes in H^+ concentration occur quickly. HCO_3^- retention and excretion are metabolic processes that are handled by the kidneys, and changes in HCO_3^- concentration take time to occur. Ultimately the traditional approach looks at either a primary respiratory or metabolic cause to determine the acid-base derangement. This may result in a respiratory acidosis or alkalosis, or a metabolic acidosis or alkalosis occurring.

Respiratory acid-base physiology

The second line of defense against acid-base disturbances is control of CO_2 concentration, achieved by ventilation of functioning lungs. Ventilation is driven, in large part by the pCO_2. Increased ventilation effectively eliminates CO_2 from the ECF, which reduces the H^+ concentration when needed. In contrast, decreased ventilation allows a build-up of CO_2, which increases the H^+ concentration within the ECF.

CO_2 is continuously formed in the body as a byproduct of the cellular metabolism of carbohydrates and fat. Approximately 10,000–15,000 mmol of CO_2 are formed each day. Once formed, it diffuses from the cells into the interstitial fluid and intravascular space. Blood flow transports CO_2 to the lungs where it diffuses into the alveoli and is then exhaled into the atmosphere by pulmonary ventilation to maintain the partial pressure of CO_2 at 40 mmHg. About 1.2 mmol/L of dissolved CO_2 is normally found within the ECF, which corresponds to a pCO_2 of about 40 mmHg (1.2 can be obtained by multiplying the solubility constant 0.03 by a measured partial pressure of 40 mmHg).

If the rate of CO_2 formation increases, the pCO_2 will also increase. If the rate of pulmonary ventilation is increased, CO_2 is blown off through the lungs and the pCO_2 will decrease. Changes in either pulmonary ventilation or the rate of CO_2 formation by the tissues can change the pCO_2. If the metabolic formation of CO_2 remains constant, the only factor affecting the pCO_2 is the rate and depth of alveolar ventilation. The more the ventilation rises, the lower the pCO_2 will fall. When CO_2 concentration increases in the presence of carbonic anhydrase, conversion to H_2CO_3 concentration increases, which corresponds to a decrease in pH. This is why CO_2 is considered a volatile acid.

Alveolar ventilation is driven by the respiratory center, which comprises several groups of neurons located bilaterally in the medulla oblongata and pons of the brain stem. The goal of respiration is to maintain relatively static concentrations of oxygen, CO_2, and H^+ in the tissues. Respiratory activity is highly responsive to changes in these variables. Excess CO_2 or H^+ in the blood act directly on the respiratory center, causing increased strength of inspiratory and expiratory motor signals. Oxygen, however, does not have a significant effect on the respiratory center of the brain, but acts on peripheral chemoreceptors located in the carotid and aortic bodies, and these transmit signals to the respiratory center for control of respiration.

When H^+ concentration increases, the pH decreases, and this causes ventilation to increase, lowering CO_2 levels, in an effort to compensate. Conversely, when H^+ concentration decreases, the pH increases, and ventilation is decreased in an effort to compensate through increasing pCO_2 levels, but not to the same degree that occurs with an increased H^+ concentration. If hypoventilation is severe enough, it may also result in less oxygen exchange and hypoxemia. In these cases the hypoxia may be the stimulus for ventilation. This limitation explains why respiratory compensation for an increased pH is never as effective as it will be for a reduction in pH, because there is a limit to how much hypercapnia and hypoxia are tolerated by the body. Respiratory control cannot completely return the pH to normal levels if a disturbance outside of the respiratory system has altered the pH. However, the respiratory system can act rapidly to minimize changes to the blood pH.

Returning to the Henderson–Hasselbalch equation, we can simplify it, and say that pH is determined by the ratio of HCO_3^- to carbon dioxide (approximated by pCO_2).

$$pH \, \alpha \, [HCO_3^- / pCO_2]$$

If pCO_2 is elevated, the kidneys will respond and attempt to compensate by increasing H^+ excretion and both preserving and generating more HCO_3^- in an effort to maintain pH balance. While respiratory changes happen quickly, the kidneys' response takes time. There may be only a mild increase in HCO_3^- concentration in an acute respiratory acidosis, but a larger response (increased HCO_3^- concentration) in a chronic respiratory acidosis.

When the primary cause of the acid-base disturbance is respiratory, the pH and pCO_2 values will change in opposite directions. When the pH is decreased (acidemia) and the pCO_2 is increased, or when the pH is increased (alkalemia) and the pCO_2 is decreased, a respiratory process is responsible for the disturbance and we know that the body's normal ventilation is somehow impaired (Figure 8.1).

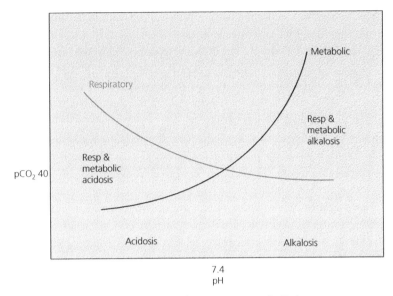

Figure 8.1 Process of acid-base balance in relation to pCO_2 and pH changes.

Respiratory acidosis

Respiratory acidosis occurs when the pH of the blood is low (acidemia) due to accumulation of, or high, pCO_2 in the blood (hypercapnia). Potential causes of respiratory acidosis include: insufficient neural drive for ventilation [e.g. anesthetics, central nervous system (CNS) disease], airway obstruction; pulmonary disease, or any disease restricting lung inflation (e.g. abdominal bloat, pleural effusion). The kidneys compensate by excreting more H^+ in the urine and reabsorbing more HCO_3^-. Because this mechanism takes a few days, there will be only a small increase in HCO_3^- concentration in acute cases but a more substantial change in cases of chronic respiratory acidosis.

If the pCO_2 is decreased, the kidneys will respond by eliminating HCO_3^- to maintain pH balance. Because the kidneys' response is slow, there may only be a slight decrease in HCO_3^- concentration in acute cases. In chronic respiratory alkalosis there will often be a more substantial change. Regardless of duration, the compensation is never complete and respiratory alkalosis (pH >7.45) will persist to some extent. This is covered in more detail in Chapter 10.

Respiratory alkalosis

Respiratory alkalosis occurs when the pH of the blood is elevated due to low CO_2 levels (hypocapnia). Potential causes include: alveolar hyperventilation, anxiety, and stimulation of the respiratory centers (i.e. from toxin ingestion, fever, or meningitis). The kidneys compensate by retaining H^+ and by excreting HCO_3^- in the urine so that blood HCO_3^- concentration is decreased in an effort to decrease the overall pH toward normal. The kidneys respond slowly, however, so this mechanism takes a few days. Typically there is only a small degree of compensation in acute cases, but a more substantial change in chronic cases.

Metabolic acid-base physiology

The third line of defense against acid-base imbalance is the kidneys. The kidneys are much slower in their response when compared to either chemical buffers or the respiratory system, but they are the most powerful of the acid-base regulatory systems. The kidneys control pH by excreting either acidic or basic urine. More specifically, the kidneys excrete and reabsorb both HCO_3^- and H^+, and generate new HCO_3^- molecules to ensure acid-base balance. For every hydrogen ion excreted, a new bicarbonate molecule is created. Renal elimination of hydrogen ions keeps the blood HCO_3^- concentration within a narrow range of 24–26 mEq/L.

Simply put, large numbers of HCO_3^- ions are filtered continuously into the renal tubules, and if these are excreted into the urine, base is lost from the blood. Large numbers of H^+ are also secreted into the tubular lumen by the tubular epithelial cells, thereby removing acid from the blood. If more H^+ is secreted than HCO_3^- ions filtered, there will be a net loss of acid from the ECF. Conversely, if more HCO_3^- ions are filtered than H^+ secreted, there will be a net loss of alkali (base).

As mentioned earlier, the body also produces non-volatile acids, including hydrochloric acid (HCl), sulfuric acid (H_2SO_4), and ammonium (NH_4), primarily from the metabolism of proteins. Renal excretion is the most significant mechanism by which these acids are removed from the body. The kidneys also have the important responsibility of preventing the loss of HCO_3^- in the urine. Under normal conditions, most of the HCO_3^- is reabsorbed from the renal tubules, thus conserving the body's primary extracellular buffer source.

H^+ secretion and reabsorption occurs in virtually all parts of the kidney's tubules except the descending and ascending thin limbs of the loop of Henle. For each HCO_3^- reabsorbed, one H^+ must be secreted. About 80% of both HCO_3^- reabsorption and H^+ secretion occurs in the proximal tubule, about 10% occurs in the thick ascending loop of Henle, and the remaining HCO_3^- flows into the distal tubules (6%) and collecting ducts (4%) (DiBartola 2012). The various renal tubular segments perform HCO_3^- reabsorption differently.

The mechanisms involved in the kidneys' regulation of acid-base are complex and can be difficult to fully understand (Figure 8.2). To simplify, we can consider these processes as being divided into a proximal tubular mechanism and a distal tubular mechanism.

The proximal tubule manages reabsorption of a majority of the HCO_3^- that was filtered through the glomerulus. It also handles production of ammonium (NH_4^+).

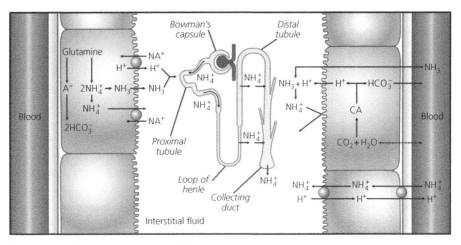

Figure 8.2 Acid-base balance in the kidneys.

H⁺ leaves the epithelial cells of the proximal tubule and enters the proximal tubule fluid by two mechanisms. The Na⁺–H⁺ antiporter, NHE3, is the primary mechanism, responsible for about one-third of this H⁺ transport. The remaining H⁺ is transported by the H⁺-adenosine triphosphatase (H⁺-ATPase) proton pump.

Filtered HCO_3^- cannot cross the membrane of the epithelial cell by simple diffusion. Instead, it combines with secreted H⁺ to produce CO_2 and H_2O. Since CO_2 is lipid-soluble, it crosses easily into the cytoplasm of the epithelial cell. Within the cell, this CO_2 combines with OH⁻ to produce HCO_3^-. The HCO_3^- then crosses the cell's basolateral membrane by a Na⁺–HCO_3^- symporter. This symporter is electrogenic, since it transfers three HCO_3^- for every one Na⁺, and this results in an imbalance in electrical charge. In contrast, the Na⁺–H⁺ antiporter in the cell's apical membrane is not electrogenic because it transfers an equal amount of charge in both directions. The basolateral membrane also has an active Na⁺–K⁺ ATPase (sodium pump) that transports three Na⁺ ions out for every two K⁺ ions that are brought into the cell. This pump is also electrogenic, but its charge imbalance is in the opposite direction to that of the Na⁺–HCO_3^- symporter. The sodium pump keeps intracellular Na⁺ low, thus creating the required Na⁺ concentration gradient to drive the H⁺–Na⁺ antiporter of the apical membrane.

The net effect of this complex and coordinated process is the reabsorption of one molecule of HCO_3^- and one molecule of Na⁺ from the tubular lumen into the bloodstream for each molecule of H⁺ secreted. Because the H⁺ is used in the reaction with the filtered HCO_3^- in the tubular lumen, no additional H⁺ is secreted from the body.

There are four major factors affecting the rate of HCO_3^- reabsorption within the proximal tubule: tubular lumen HCO_3^- concentration, tubular lumen flow rate, arterial pCO_2, and angiotensin II levels. An increase in any of these factors can cause an increase in HCO_3^- reabsorption. Although there is no net excretion of H+ from the body, the proximal tubular mechanism is extremely important in acid-base regulation because the loss of HCO_3^- has an acidifying effect.

The mechanism for H^+ secretion in the proximal tubule is described as high capacity because it removes the vast majority of the daily fixed acid load, and low gradient because it cannot decrease the pH by very much (maximum change of only 0.4–0.9).

Excretion of ammonium (NH_4^+) by the kidneys is essential for eliminating the daily fixed acid load and regenerating HCO_3^-. Most of the NH_4^+ to be excreted is produced within the proximal tubular cells. NH_4^+ produced is from glutamine, which enters the cell both from the capillaries around the tubules (80%) and from the filtrate (20%), with action from the enzyme glutaminase. Additional ammonium is produced when the glutamate is metabolized to produce alpha-ketoglutarate. This molecule contains two negatively charged carboxylate groups, so further metabolism of it within the cell results in the production of two HCO_3^- anions. This occurs if it is oxidized to CO_2, or if it is metabolized to glucose.

About 75% of the ammonium produced within the proximal tubule is removed from the tubular fluid within the renal medulla so that the amount of ammonium entering the distal tubule is small. Most of the NH_4^+ is involved in cycling within the medulla. About 75% of the proximally produced NH_4^+ is removed from the tubular fluid in the medulla so that the amount of NH_4^+ entering the distal tubule is small. The thick ascending limb of the loop of Henle is the important segment for removing NH_4^+. Some of the interstitial NH_4^+ returns to the late proximal tubule and reenters the medulla (where it is recycled).

If the ammonium returns to the bloodstream, it is metabolized in the liver to urea (Krebs–Henseleit cycle) with net production of one hydrogen ion per NH_4^+ molecule.

In contrast to the proximal tubular mechanism described above, the distal tubule provides a low-capacity, high-gradient system. It accounts for a much lower excretion of the daily acid load, but can achieve a pH reduction of considerable magnitude (up to three units).

Specific processes that take place in the distal tubule are the formation of titratable acidity (TA), addition of NH_4^+ to the luminal fluid, and reabsorption of any remaining HCO_3^-.

H^+ is produced from CO_2 and H_2O (just as it was in the proximal tubular cells), and it is actively transported into the distal tubular lumen by an H^+-ATPase pump. TA represents the H^+ that is buffered mostly by phosphate, which is present in significant concentration. Creatinine may also contribute to TA. If ketoacids are present, they also contribute to TA. In severe diabetic ketoacidosis, beta-hydroxybutyrate is the major ketoacid component of TA. The TA can be measured in the urine from the amount of sodium hydroxide needed to titrate the urine pH back to 7.4, hence the term "titratable acidity."

As mentioned, NH_4^+ is predominantly produced by proximal tubular cells. Medullary cycling maintains high medullary interstitial concentrations of NH_4^+

and low distal tubule fluid concentrations. The lower the urine pH, the greater the amount of NH_4^+ that is transferred from the medullary interstitium into the medullary collecting duct as it passes through the medulla to the renal pelvis.

NH_4^+ is not measured as part of the TA, because the high pK of NH_4 means no H^+ is removed from NH_4^+ during titration to a pH of 7.4. NH_4^+ excretion is extremely important in increasing acid excretion in systemic acidosis; it can and does increase markedly in this situation. NH_4^+ excretion increases as urine pH falls and this effect is dramatically increased in acidosis. Formation of NH_4^+ prevents further fall in pH as the pKa of the reaction is so high.

Normally, the entire filtered load of HCO_3^- is reabsorbed: 80% in the proximal tubule, 10% in the thick ascending limb of the loop of Henle, 6% in the distal tubule, and 4% in the collecting duct. There is an increase in the HCO_3^- concentration due to a reduced volume of filtrate as water is removed in the loop of Henle. HCO_3^- reabsorption in the thick ascending limb of the loop of Henle occurs by similar mechanisms as in the proximal tubule. That is: apical Na^+–H^+ antiport, basolateral Na^+–HCO_3^- symport, and Na^+–K^+ ATPase. HCO_3^- reabsorption here is stimulated by the presence of luminal furosemide. The cells in this part of the tubule also contain carbonic anhydrase, which helps facilitate the production of H_2O and CO_2 from luminal carbonic acid.

Any amount of HCO_3^- entering the distal tubule can be reabsorbed. The distal tubule has a limited capacity to reabsorb HCO_3^-, and if the filtered load is high and a large amount is delivered distally there will be net HCO_3^- excretion. The process of HCO_3^- reabsorption in the distal tubule is somewhat different from in the proximal tubule: H^+ secretion by the intercalated cells in the distal collecting duct involves a H^+-ATPase, and HCO_3^- transfer across the basolateral membrane involves a HCO_3^-–Cl^- exchanger.

Excretion of one H^+ results in the return of one HCO_3^- and one Na^+ to the bloodstream. HCO_3^- effectively replaces the acid anion which is excreted in the urine. The net acid excretion in the urine is equal to the sum of the TA and NH_4^+ concentration minus the HCO_3^- concentration (if present in the urine). The H^+ concentration accounts for only a very small amount of the H^+ excretion.

When derangements occur and the changes in pH and in pCO_2 are in the same direction, a metabolic process is the cause. When the pH is decreased and the pCO_2 is decreased, or when the pH is elevated and the pCO_2 is elevated, a metabolic process is responsible for the disturbance and we know that the body's normal metabolism is somehow impaired.

The liver is important, but often overlooked, in acid-base physiology. It is a metabolically active organ that may be either a significant net producer or consumer of H^+ ions. The amounts of acid involved may be very large. The liver is responsible for: CO_2 production from complete oxidation of substrates, metabolism of organic acid anions (such as lactate, ketones and amino acids), metabolism of NH_4^+, and production of plasma proteins (particularly albumin).

Metabolic alkalosis

In metabolic alkalosis, the increased HCO_3^- level will result in increased filtration of HCO_3^-, provided the glomerular filtration rate (GFR) has not decreased. The kidney is usually very efficient at excreting excess HCO_3^-, but this capacity can be impaired in certain circumstances.

Referring back to our simplified equation:

$$pH \; \alpha \; [HCO_3^- / pCO_2]$$

If there is an increase in $[HCO_3^-]$, the body will try to retain CO_2 to maintain pH balance. This compensation also happens quickly, but again the compensation is not complete, so some degree of metabolic alkalemia (pH >7.45) persists.

In metabolic alkalosis the low pH is either due to a gain in HCO_3^- or a loss in H^+. Potential causes include: iatrogenic, from ingestion or administration of HCO_3^-, or vomiting, due to a loss of gastric acid (especially in pyloric obstruction or high duodenal obstruction). There is often little in the way of respiratory compensation to metabolic alkalosis. Respiratory compensation would require slower or shallower breathing which would potentially compromise oxygen saturation levels (pO_2). However, the kidneys will respond over time with increased HCO_3^- excretion into the ECF and increased H^+ reabsorption.

Metabolic acidosis

In metabolic acidosis the low pH is either from a gain in acid (other than H_2CO_3) or from the loss of bicarbonate. Potential causes include: renal failure, as HCO_3^- is not being returned to the ECF; diabetes mellitus with production of ketone bodies, which are weak acids; inadequate circulation (e.g. cardiac disease, shock), which can lead to tissue hypoxia; and anaerobic metabolism, which produces lactic acid; and diarrhea, with loss of HCO_3^- from alkaline intestinal fluids. The respiratory system begins to compensate for metabolic acidosis within minutes to hours by increasing the ventilation rate. With severe chronic metabolic acidosis (such as ketoacidosis), animals may develop a deep, labored breathing pattern (Kussmaul respiration) instead of tachypnea. Providing that the cause of the acidosis is not due to renal insufficiency, the kidneys will also respond to a metabolic acidosis by increasing H^+ excretion and increasing reabsorption of HCO_3^-. This response takes a few days to develop.

If there is a decrease in $[HCO_3^-]$, the body will respond as outlined above, by decreasing the pCO_2 in an effort to minimize the change in body pH. This response happens almost immediately; the patient simply breathes faster (i.e. ventilation rate is increased) to rid the body of excess CO_2. Typically, the compensation is not complete, so there will still be some degree of metabolic acidemia (pH <7.35).

Blood gas measurement

An ABG analyzer measures the pH and levels of both oxygen and carbon dioxide in the blood from an artery. This testing is used to determine acid-base balance, and also assess how well the patient's lungs are performing.

The most important values in ABG analysis, utilizing the traditional approach, are pH, PCO_2 and HCO_3^-. Most blood gas analyzers directly measure pH and pCO_2, and calculate the HCO_3^- concentration. CO_2 concentration results vary considerably depending on factors associated with sample collection, handling, timing, and the specific equipment used for analysis. Each of these factors is of critical importance and can affect the accuracy of pH and CO_2 measurements.

Venous samples can also be used for blood gas evaluation, but there is a significant difference in the value for pO_2 between venous and arterial samples. The venous sample normally has a much lower value than the arterial sample. pCO_2 is expected to be slightly higher in venous blood, and venous pH is generally lower. ABG may not show an accurate acid-base status in peripheral tissues, so venous samples should be obtained from a central vessel whenever possible (Table 8.2).

The anion gap

Anion gap (AG) is another useful tool for analyzing a patient's acid-base status (Figure 8.3). To maintain electroneutrality within the ECF, the sum of the concentrations of the positively charged ions (cations) must equal that of the negatively charged ions (anions). Cations that we typically measure are sodium (Na^+) and potassium (K^+). Other, often unmeasured, cations such as calcium (Ca^{++}) and magnesium (Mg^{++}) are present in much lower concentrations and are not used in the calculation of AG. Measured anions are chloride (Cl^-) and bicarbonate (HCO_3^-). There are many unmeasured anions, including blood proteins, phosphates, and sulfates.

The AG is the difference between the measured cations and the measured anions. As an example, let us suppose we have:

$$\left[K^+\right] = 4, \left[Na^+\right] = 140, \left[Cl^-\right] = 100, \left[HCO_3^-\right] = 24$$

Table 8.2 Normal arterial and venous acid-base values for cats and dogs

	pH	CO_2	HCO_3^-	BE	AG
Dog arterial	7.35–7.45	35–45	22–27	–2 to +2	12–20
Dog venous	7.32–7.5	33–50	18–26	–2 to +2	12–20
Cat arterial	7.24–7.45	25–37	15–22	–2 to +2.5	12–18
Cat venous	7.28–7.41	33–45	18–23	–2 to 2.5	12–18

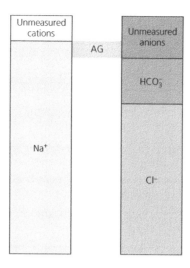

Figure 8.3 The anion gap.

That gives us a total of 144 cations ($[Na^+]+[K^+]$), and a total of 124 anions ($[Cl^-]+[HCO_3^-]$). The difference between cations and anions is 20 ($144-124$). Since potassium is present in such a small number compared to the other ions, it is typically left out of the equation altogether:

$$AG=\left[Na^+\right]-\left[Cl^-+HCO_3^-\right]$$

Using the previous example, the AG would be $140-[100+24]=16$. In dogs, a normal range for AG is 12–20. In cats, the normal range is 12–18. This gap, or difference, refers to the presence of unmeasured anions. The primary unmeasured anion is protein, or more specifically albumin. If the concentration of unmeasured anions increases, then Cl^- and HCO_3^- will decrease to maintain electrolyte balance, and the AG will increase. The AG can usually be approximated by multiplying the serum albumin concentration by a factor of 3. Potential causes of an increased AG are: lactic acidosis, ketoacidosis, kidney failure with increased sulfates and phosphates, uremia, and ethylene glycol intoxication.

Base excess

Base excess (BE) is another value used in determining the nature of acid-base disturbances. It was introduced in 1958 by Poul Astrup and Ole Siggaard-Andersen as a measure of treatment required to correct metabolic disturbances (Astrup, P. & Severinghaus 1986). The "in-vitro" BE, however, is dependent on hemoglobin level, and was the subject of some debate.

A BE refers to the amount of strong acid that must be added to each liter of fully oxygenated blood to return the pH to 7.4 at a temperature of 37 °C and a pCO_2 of 40 mmHg. A base deficit (also viewed as a negative BE) refers to the amount of a strong base that must be added to each liter of fully oxygenated blood to return the pH to 7.4 at a temperature of 37 °C and a pCO_2 of 40 mmHg. The normal range for BE is –2 to +2 mEq. BE is only affected by non-volatile (fixed) acids, and therefore a value outside of the normal range suggests a metabolic cause for an acid-base disturbance. In general, a negative value, or base deficit (<=–3), suggests a metabolic acidosis, and a positive value (>=3) indicates a metabolic alkalosis.

BE can be estimated by the following equation:

$$BE = 0.93 \left[HCO_3 - 24.4 + 14.8 \left(pH - 7.4 \right) \right]$$

or

$$BE = 0.93 \times HCO_3 + 13.77 \times pH - 124.58$$

BE can be helpful in indicating the metabolic nature of a disorder, but it can also be misleading. An alkalemia or acidemia may be primary or secondary to respiratory acidosis or alkalosis. The BE does not take into account the appropriateness of the metabolic response for any given disorder, and this limits its utility when interpreting results.

Process of acid-base analysis

How does all this information apply to an actual patient? The following four areas should be considered when evaluating acid-base results:

1 Is there an acid-base disturbance present?
2 What is the primary problem?
3 Is there an expected compensatory response? Or is there a mixed disturbance?
4 What underlying disease(s) is/are causing the problem?

Make a habit to approach acid-base analysis step by step, in the same way, every time. Working through it in a systematic way will make it less likely to miss an important finding. Be sure to think of the following (Figure 8.4):

- Is there an acid-base disturbance present?
  - What is the pH? Normal? High? Low?
  - Is the sample acidotic? Alkalotic? Or normal?
- What is the HCO_3^-?
  - Normal? High? Low?
- What is the PCO_2?
  - What is the ventilatory status? Hyperventilating? Hypoventilating? Normal?
- What is the primary problem?
  - Which abnormal result is causing the derangement to the pH?
  - Is the problem primarily metabolic or respiratory?

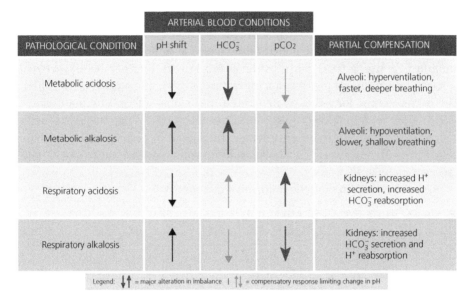

Figure 8.4 Arterial blood gases chart. (Source: Courtesy of Robert Thorp.)

- Is there an expected compensatory response? Or a mixed problem?
  - Evaluate secondary derangements: are they within compensatory levels? (Remember the body will not over compensate!)
- Evaluate underlying disease in deciding course of treatment for acid-base derangement and treat accordingly.

Tips and tricks for acid-base

Most people have a difficult time not becoming confused when evaluating acid-base assessments. Therefore some helpful tips are necessary! Both of the following tips are widely known in the human nursing profession.

Tip 1: Mnemonic: R.O.M.E.

$$R = Respiratory$$
$$O = Opposite$$
$$M = Metabolic$$
$$E = Equal$$

This tip helps you remember which way derangements go (up or down), if it is due to a metabolic or respiratory cause (Figure 8.4). In the respiratory side of acid-base the arrows go opposite (if pH is high, CO_2 is low). Metabolic acid-base changes are equal (if pH is low, bicarb is low).

Tip 2: Acid-base tic-tac-toe

Yes, acid-base can be as simple as playing tic-tac-toe. Normals for all values are needed in order to utilize these charts. In this chart there are three columns: acid/acidic, normal, and alkaline/basic (Figure 8.5).

The values for pH, HCO_3^-, and pCO_2 are needed for this chart. Determine whether each value is high, normal, or low and insert it into the column that applies. For example:

- pH: 7.1 is low, therefore it is acidic and would go in the acid column.
- HCO_3^-: 10 is low, therefore it would go in the acid column.
- PCO_2: 24 is low, therefore it would go in the alkaline column.

The chart would then look like Figure 8.6.

Next, match it up by determining which column matches with the pH. In this case the pH is in the acid column, so there is an acidosis. Then determine which parameter is also in the acid column. In this example it is HCO_3^-. Since HCO_3^- is metabolic, it becomes clear there is a metabolic acidosis. Since the pCO_2 is under the alkaline column, the change in pH is clearly not caused by the respiratory side. However, since the pH is abnormal, it can be determined there is compensation occurring on the respiratory side. So there is a metabolic acidosis with

ACID	NORMAL	ALKALINE

Figure 8.5 Tic-tac-toe method of determining acid-base imbalance. (Source: Based on http://nurselabs.com)

ACID	NORMAL	ALKALINE
pH^- 7.1		pCO_2^- 24
HCO_3^- 10		

Figure 8.6 How to use the tic-tac-toe method to determine acid-base imbalance.

respiratory compensation. If the pCO_2 had been normal, there would be a metabolic acidosis with no respiratory compensation.

These tips can help determine basic acid-base changes and their cause. Assessment of oxygenation will be covered in a later chapter of this book.

Summary

As discussed, the body attempts to regulate blood pH within the narrow range of 7.35 and 7.45. This is achieved primarily by the lungs and the kidneys, and to some extent the liver, employing bicarbonate and other buffers. Primary changes in bicarbonate signal a metabolic disorder, and primary changes in carbon dioxide are respiratory in nature. Disorders of acid-base balance can lead to severe complications in many disease states. While they can be life threatening, they are usually secondary to a disease state, and the clinical condition of the patient should be appropriately assessed.

There is an acid-base imbalance when the pH is less than 7.35: this is termed an acidosis; or when the pH is above 7.45: this is an alkalosis. If the value pCO_2, which is normally 40 mmHg, has moved in the same direction as the pH, the primary cause for the disturbance is metabolic; if it has moved in the opposite direction from the pH, the primary cause is respiratory.

Mnemonics or easy ways to chart acid-base results can be helpful for quickly determining the underlying acid-base imbalance in a patient, which in turn can aid in pinpointing the underlying cause or disease and treatments needed.

References

Astrup, P. & Severinghaus, J. W. (1986). *The History of Blood Gases, Acids and Bases*. Copenhagen, Denmark: Munksgaard.

DiBartola, S. P. (ed.), (2012). *Fluid, Electrolyte and Acid-Base Disorders in Small Animal Practice*, 4th ed. St. Louis, MO: Elsevier Saunders.

Hess, D. R., MacIntyre, N. R., Mishoe, S. C., & Galvin, W. F. (2012). *Respiratory Care: Principles and Practice*, 2nd ed. Sudbury, MA: Jones and Bartlett Learning.

Po, H. N. & Shenozan, N. M. (2001). The Henderson–Hasselbalch equation: Its history and limitations. *Journal of Chemical Education* **78**(11).

Preston, R. (2011) *Acid-Base, Fluids, and Electrolytes made ridiculously simple*, 2nd ed. Miami, FL: MedMaster, Inc.

Rose, D. B. & Post, T. W. (2001). *Clinical Physiology of Acid-Base and Electrolyte Disorders*, 5th ed. New York: McGraw-Hill.

Stewart, P. A. (1981). *How to Understand Acid-Base: A quantitative acid-base primer for biology and medicine*. New York/Oxford: Elsevier.

Stewart, P. A. (1983). Modern quantitative acid-base chemistry. *Canadian Journal of Physiology and Pharmacology* **61**.

CHAPTER 9
Metabolic Blood Gas Disorders

Eric Zamora-Moran, MBA, RVT, VTS (Anesthesia & Analgesia)

Veterinary technicians are often the first line of defense when it comes to patient care. They are the first members of the veterinary staff to evaluate, triage, and perform a medical examination of the patient. Technicians are faced each day with a variety of emergent conditions, and some may be life-threatening and in need of immediate care. As the first medical staff members to evaluate our patients, their examination must be thorough and directed at the complaint. A variety of clinical parameters should be considered when evaluating a patient for treatment. These include signalment, vital signs, mentation, ventilation, and perfusion. Acquisition of pertinent information from the patient's owner must be obtained for the veterinarian in charge, as he or she will ultimately make the decision to place the patient at the head of the line or to delay the patient's examination in favor of treating a patient with a condition of greater urgency. A structured assessment of all parameters, including developing or current disorders of acid-base balance, may result in a better outcome for your patient.

Acid-base review pertaining to metabolic blood gas disorders

To understand the acid-base homeostasis and disorders related to acid-base derangements, it is necessary to understand the variety of homeostatic mechanisms that maintain acid-base balance in the blood. If the pH becomes too high or too low, proteins and cells in the body will denature and will be unable to function properly.

Acid-Base and Electrolyte Handbook for Veterinary Technicians, First Edition.
Edited by Angela Randels-Thorp and David Liss.
© 2017 John Wiley & Sons, Inc. Published 2017 by John Wiley & Sons, Inc.
Companion website: www.wiley.com/go/liss/electrolytes

pH and hydrogen ion concentration

pH can be easily described in three words: power of hydrogen. pH has an inverse relationship with hydrogen ion concentration (H^+) and is often compared to the most common neutral fluid on earth: water (H_2O). The relationship between pH and hydrogen ion concentration is defined in the Henderson–Hasselbalch equation:

$$pH = pK_a + \log \frac{[A^-]}{[HA]}$$

There is an inverse relationship between pH and hydrogen ion concentration. As the hydrogen ion (H^+) concentration increases, the pH becomes lower. An acidic pH is considered lower than 7.35 and represents an increase in hydrogen ion concentration above normal. Lower concentrations of hydrogen ions will result in an alkaline pH, which refers to a pH of over 7.45.

Normal physiologic pH is typically between 7.35 and 7.45 (DiBartola 2012). The body controls pH through a variety of homeostatic mechanisms. These include the use of physiologic buffers to prevent an imbalance that would result in an acidemia or alkalemia. A normal pH reading on a particular patient *does not necessarily rule out a metabolic acid-base disorder.* It simply means that the overall blood pH is neither too acidic (acidemia) nor too alkalotic (alkalemia). The body has compensatory mechanisms that work to correct variations in ph. Mixed disorders resulting in a neutral pH can also occur. These mechanisms will be discussed in detail in Chapter 11. Briefly, exchange of carbon dioxide and oxygen in the lungs can aid in compensating to restore the physiologic pH to near normal within minutes through changes in rate of breathing. In the lungs, the exchange of carbon dioxide for oxygen is a major mechanism for short-term correction of pH. pH will increase or become more alkaline within minutes as CO_2 concentration decreases in response to hyperventilation. Conversely, the pH will decrease or become more acidic as CO_2 levels increase (Battaglia 2007). Accumulation of excess CO_2 occurs when respirations are depressed and ventilation is impaired. Over several days, the kidneys can also help restore balance by excretion or retention of hydrogen ions and/or bicarbonate as a compensatory mechanism for the respiratory system. The kidneys' response is slower than that of the lungs, however, and are therefore not as efficient in compensating for respiratory derangements.

Calculating pH (Henderson–Hasselbalch method)

$$pH = \frac{HCO_3^-}{\alpha pCO_2}$$

$\alpha = CO_2$ solubility coefficient of 0.03

(Irizarry & Reiss 2009)

Hydrogen ions are an acid formed as a byproduct of cellular metabolism. At a normal pH of 7.4, the level of H^+ is 40 nEq/L (0.00000040 g-atoms/L). H^+ levels have a direct effect on the pH level. If H^+ doubles (80 nEq/L), pH decreases by 0.3 units. Thus if H^+ increased by four times (160 nEq/L), the pH would decrease by 0.6 units, resulting in a pH of 6.8. If the H^+ were at half the normal amount (20 nEq/L), the pH would increase to 7.7 units (DiBartola 2012).

Buffer

The body regulates pH within a tight framework through a variety of complex buffering systems. Buffers include combinations of weak acids and a conjugate base with accompanying salts. A chemical reaction between the buffer and hydrogen ions regulate changes in hydrogen ion concentration to maintain physiologic pH under normal circumstances. Therefore, buffers aid in neutralizing strong acids or combine with bases by exchanging protons or ions. Bicarbonate is a well-known buffer type, but pH is also maintained by a variety of non-bicarbonate buffers (Figure 9.1). Bicarbonate works as the primary buffer in the extracellular fluid (ECF). Non-bicarbonate buffers, including proteins and phosphates, are the primary buffers in intracellular fluid (DiBartola 2012). The addition of a strong acid to a buffer will cause the dissociation of protons from the acid, which will then combine with the salt of the buffer, limiting the change in pH. The body is continually converting CO_2, H_2O, H^+, and HCO_3^- to maintain pH within normal ranges. The following equation represents this interaction (Reece 2009):

$$CO_2 + H_2O \leftrightarrow H^+ + HCO_3^-$$

The following is an example of sodium bicarbonate buffering an acid, resulting in a weaker acid and a salt (Reece 2009):

$$HCL + NaHCO_3^- \rightarrow H_2CO_3 + NaCl$$

Below is an example of carbonic acid (weak acid) buffering sodium hydroxide base:

$$NaOH + H_2CO_3 \rightarrow NaHCO_3^- + H_2O$$

Bicarbonate is considered one of the most important buffers in the body and it also contributes to coagulation, cardiac function, and neuromuscular function (Thomas & Lerche 2011). Ninety percent of the carbon dioxide produced by

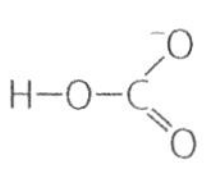

Figure 9.1 Bicarbonate ion (HCO_3^-).

metabolism is carried in the blood in the form of bicarbonate as it is converted as illustrated in the above equation. It is freely filtered by the kidney and can be excreted when needed or reabsorbed to neutralize acids—whichever the body needs at any given time.

Non-bicarbonate buffers include proteins, inorganic, and organic phosphates that primarily serve as buffers in the intracellular space. Bone provides an additional large source of buffer in the form of calcium carbonate and calcium phosphate. Up to 40% of buffering can be done from these resources found in bone. In the blood, proteins such as hemoglobin are an important component of the body's buffering intracellular buffering system. Plasma proteins only account for 20% of the body's buffering capacity.

Buffer systems may be either a closed or open system. The body's buffering system is an open system. In an open buffering system, the weak acid and conjugate base can be independently controlled. In the body, this refers to independent elimination of carbon dioxide through changes in respiration, increasing the body's capacity to deal with significant changes in pH through compensatory efforts of the opposite system. A closed buffering system would not allow for such compensation to occur as a reciprocal action would have to occur in the other system. By definition a closed system refers to a fixed amount of a buffer in solution which can be depleted as hydrogen ions are added to the solution.

Base excess

Base excess (BE), by definition, is the quantity of acid or base required to continuously change and maintain 1 L of blood to pH of 7.4 at 37 °C and a pCO_2 of 40 mmHg (DiBartola 2012). It refers to the amount of acid or hydrogen ions required to return the blood pH to normal if the pCO_2 is adjusted to normal (de Morais & DiBartola 2008). This particular definition is not always helpful in clinical practice. Clinically, the measurement of BE can be useful, however, for determination of the patient's overall acid-base status. A negative BE is reflecting an acid excess, confirming presence of an acidemia. Alternatively, a positive value BE is supportive of an alkalemia. BE is a useful tool for evaluation of patients with mixed disorders (see Chapter 11).

CO_2

CO_2 is another byproduct of cellular metabolism. The lungs primarily regulate CO_2, as CO_2 levels are the primary determinant of the respiratory drive. Peripheral chemoreceptors in the body sense the level of carbon dioxide in arterial blood. When carbon dioxide crosses the blood–brain barrier and forms hydrogen ions, central chemoreceptors signal the brain to contract the diaphragm to produce respiration and gas exchange at the alveolar level. CO_2 is transported through the blood in three ways: 20–30% is bound to hemoglobin within red blood cells, 5–10% is dissolved in plasma, and 60–70% is turned into carbonic acid in presence of carbonic anhydrase. Carbonic acid is a weak acid in equilibrium with bicarbonate in the blood. When both are present, a buffer system is formed and can be described by the following equation:

$$H_2CO_3 + H_2O = H_3O^+ + HCO_3^-$$

Normally, the ratio of bicarbonate to carbonic acid is 20:1. Normal metabolism results in the production of more acid than base, but the high bicarbonate content of the buffering system is able to readily neutralize metabolic acid. Carbonic acid is unstable in aqueous solution and decomposes to form water and carbon dioxide which can then be expired by the lungs (Thomas & Lerche 2011):

$$CO_2 + H_2O = H_2CO_3$$

CO_2 levels may be measured in venous or arterial blood samples as the partial pressure of carbon dioxide (pCO_2), or by capnography if the patient is intubated. The normal partial pressure of carbon dioxide in the arterial blood is between 35 and 45 mmHg. Venous samples will have a slightly higher pCO_2 reading but can be an adequate way to evaluate ventilator status of a particular patient. Capnography is a measurement of end-tidal carbon dioxide ($ETCO_2$) obtained by instrumentation attached to the end of a tracheal tube and is also measured in mmHg (Bryant 2013). $ETCO_2$ is approximately 38 mmHg (35–45 mmHg) at an atmospheric pressure of 760 mmHg. The difference between $PaCO_2$ and $ETCO_2$ is known as the CO_2 gradient.

Anion gap

Though the name may sound like an abnormality, calculating the anion gap can be useful to consider when determining the etiology of an acid-base disorder. "Anion gap" refers to the difference between the total concentrations of measured cations and the concentrations of measured anions. Measured cations include sodium, calcium, potassium, and magnesium (DiBartola 2012). Measured anions include chloride, bicarbonate, phosphate, sulfate, lactate, organic acids, and proteins. The anion gap is calculated using the following formula:

Anion gap calculation

$$\left(Na^+ + K^+\right) - \left(Cl^- + HCO_3^-\right)$$

If potassium levels are normal, potassium ions will have little effect on the anion gap. The anion gap is calculated by the following simplified formula:

$$Na^+ - \left(Cl^- + HCO_3^-\right)$$

Normal AG is 12–24 mEq/L in dogs and 13–27 mEq/L in cats. An elevated anion gap is usually a result of a decrease in bicarbonate levels and metabolic acidosis (Norkus 2012). If a normal anion gap exists with a metabolic acidosis, an increase in chloride occurs as the kidney works to compensate and these patients have a hyperchloremic metabolic acidosis (Norkus 2012) according to the traditional approach to acid-base. An increased anion gap may also be seen in older patients (DiBartola 2012). If the pH of a patient is normal with a high anion gap, this is suggestive of acidosis. These patients likely have a mixed disorder resulting in the normal pH level. There is a mnemonic to remember the common causes of increased anion gap metabolic acidosis: MUDPILES. It represents methanol, uremia, diabetic ketoacidosis, propylene glycol, iron, isoniazid, lactic acidosis, ethylene glycol, and salicylates.

Temperature

Temperature has a direct effect on acid-base balance in the body. Ionization normally increases with temperature in any ionizable system, so the amount of active hydrogen ions active in a solution usually increases with increased temperature, resulting in a lower pH. As the pH decreases, the respiratory rate will increase to compensate. Most blood gas values are based on normal body temperatures of 37 °C (98.6 °F). Some machines will allow entry of the patient's current body temperature when running arterial blood gas samples. This may be useful to do in patients that are either hypo- or hyperthermic.

Simple versus mixed acid-base disorders

When diagnosing an acid-base disturbance, it is essential to determine if the disorder is a simple or a more complex, mixed disorder. A mixed acid-base disorder should not be confused with a simple or mixed disorder with a compensatory response. Simple acid-base disturbances are typically associated with a primary disorder, followed by a secondary compensatory response (Battaglia 2007). The compensatory response is usually predictable, which allows the clinician to determine if the compensation is appropriate or if there is a mixed disorder. A mixed acid-base disturbance refers to two primary and unassociated disturbances occurring together. It is important to differentiate a mixed disorder from compensatory mechanisms, as accurate diagnosis may allow early detection of potential complications that can guide treatment. Compensation of metabolic disturbances is discussed in the next section of this chapter.

A patient who is suffering from either metabolic acidosis or metabolic alkalosis is a patient who has a simple acid-base disorder. These patients will demonstrate either an acidemia or alkalemia, respectively (DiBartola 2012). An example of a simple acid-base disorder is a patient who has a significant loss of potassium due to the frequent administration of a loop diuretic. It is well known that potassium and acid-base balance are linked. In general, acidemia is associated with an increase in the plasma concentration of potassium, thought to be the result of potassium moving to the ECF in exchange for hydrogen ions. The reverse occurs with alkalosis.

An easy way to differentiate between a simple and a mixed acid-base disorder is by comparison of the response of the patient to the predicted compensatory response. According to the traditional approach, a patient with a metabolic acidosis has a primary decrease in bicarbonate. The body's response is hyperventilation and the expected compensatory decrease in pCO_2 is 1.2 mmHg for every 1 mmol/L decrease in HCO_3^-. In patients with respiratory acidosis or alkalosis, the mechanism of compensation is retention or excretion of HCO_3^- by the kidney. Typically acute respiratory acidosis causes a compensatory increase in HCO_3^- of 0.15 mEq/L for every 1 mmHg elevation in pCO_2 (DiBartola 2012). Patients with chronic respiratory acidosis compensate over several days by retaining HCO_3^- in the kidneys. The expected increase in HCO_3^- is 0.35 mEq/L for every 1 mmHg increase in pCO_2 (DiBartola 2012). In patients with acute respiratory alkalosis, the HCO_3^- will decrease by 0.25 mEq/L for every 1 mmHg decrease in pCO_2 (DiBartola 2012). In a patient with chronic respiratory alkalosis a decrease is noted in HCO_3^- by 0.55 mEq/L for every 1 mmHg in pCO_2 (DiBartola 2012). It may take the kidneys up to one week to reach maximal compensation in order to correct the blood pH (DiBartola 2012). As noted in the text, during respiratory blood gas disorders, the relationship or ratio of HCO_3^- per pCO_2 is greater in chronic cases.

If the derangements in an acid-base disorder appear to be within the range of an expected compensatory response, it is most likely a simple acid-base disorder with compensation, either partial or complete. If the disturbances appear to be unrelated and are not within expected ranges for compensation, a mixed acid-base disturbance is likely. Mixed disorders are discussed in more detail in Chapter 11.

Compensatory responses

In addition to the use of buffers to modulate pH balance, the body reacts to acid-base derangements with a compensatory response, which allows maintenance of physiologic pH. The lungs control the level of CO_2 by hypoventilation or hyperventilation. This compensatory response occurs in minutes. In patients with metabolic acidosis, the expected respiratory compensatory response is a decrease of 1.2 mmHg in pCO_2 for every 1 mEq/L decrease in HCO_3^- (DiBartola 2012). This is achieved by hyperventilation. In patients with metabolic alkalosis, the expected respiratory compensatory response is an increase in the pCO_2 of 0.6 mmHg for every 1 mEq/L increase in HCO_3^- (DiBartola 2012). This is achieved by decreased respirations. The respiratory compensatory response attempts to bring the pH to normal by normalizing the HCO_3^- : pCO_2 ratio (Irizarry & Reiss 2009). The pH will typically still reflect the primary metabolic blood gas disorder present, however (Figure 9.2). In a primary respiratory acid-base disturbance, the kidneys will compensate over several days to retain HCO_3^- or to increase HCO_3^- secretion to restore a neutral pH.

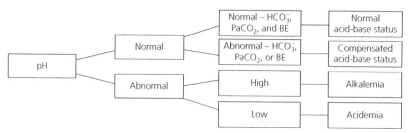

Figure 9.2 Flowchart indicating normal versus compensated acid-base disturbances and alkalemia versus acidemia.

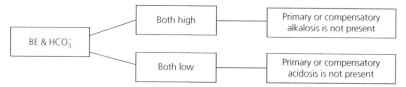

Figure 9.3 Flowchart indicating when primary and compensatory alkalosis or acidosis is not present.

If a compensatory response is not noted, or a neutral pH is seen, a mixed acid-base disorder should be suspected. It is always important to remember that compensatory responses will never overcompensate for a primary blood gas disorder (Figure 9.3; Waddell 2013). If overcompensation occurs, a mixed disorder should be suspected (see Chapter 11).

Metabolic alkalosis

Pathophysiology

Metabolic alkalosis, according to the traditional approach, is a primary increase in serum bicarbonate concentration that will occur in any condition associated with excessive retention or resorption of HCO_3^- or loss of hydrogen ions. Metabolic alkalosis may also occur as the result of an excessive loss of chloride (Cl^-) or after administration of a base ($NaHCO_3^-$) (Norkus 2012). Iatrogenic metabolic alkalosis due to administration of a base is uncommon, but may result from overzealous administration of $NaHCO_3^-$ or phosphorus binders (DiBartola 2012).

The level of urine chloride can aid to classify the causes of metabolic alkalosis, although both types of metabolic alkalosis can coexist in the same patient. Chloride-responsive metabolic alkalosis refers to alkalosis with a urine chloride concentration of less than 20 mEq/L. These patients are typically hypochloremic as well. Chloride-responsive metabolic alkalosis is the most common form of metabolic alkalosis and it is termed "chloride-responsive" because it usually can be corrected after IV administration of NaCl. One common cause of chloride-responsive metabolic alkalosis is volume depletion, which results in a stimulus for increased reabsorption of HCO_3^- by the kidney. Another important cause and consequence of metabolic alkalosis is hypokalemia. Hypokalemia and hypomagnesemia cause excretion of hydrogen due to reabsorption of potassium and magnesium in the kidney. Hypokalemia results in increased retention of HCO_3^- by the kidney.

Loop diuretics and thiazide diuretics are both causes of chloride-responsive alkalosis. Diuretic therapy may initially cause an elevation of serum chloride by acting on the sodium-potassium-chloride co-transporter in the thick ascending limb of the loop of Henle. This inhibits chloride reabsorption by competitive binding to the Cl^- binding site. After chloride stores are depleted, the urine chloride concentration will fall to <25 mEq/L. The loss of fluid from excretion of sodium results in what is called a contraction alkalosis. This refers to the loss of water in the extracellular space. This fluid loss is poor in bicarbonate and rich in chloride. Since the kidneys subsequently retain bicarbonate, the increased bicarbonate concentration reacts with additional hydrogen ions, raising the pH. With contraction of volume that occurs, the original amount of bicarbonate is dissolved in a smaller amount of fluid, thereby increasing the overall concentration of bicarbonate until the patient's volume has been restored.

Excessive loss of Cl^- is frequently the result of vomiting. Patients who are vomiting lose large amounts of chloride in the form of hydrochloric acid from gastric acid. They also lose potassium and sodium, which causes the kidneys to compensate by retention of sodium in the collecting system in exchange for hydrogen ions, which results in an overall loss, or decrease, of $[H^+]$. Gastric loss of hydrogen ions can also occur after nasogastric suctioning or due to some forms of diarrhea. A decrease in gastric acid results in hypochloremic metabolic alkalosis, which is sometimes associated with gastric foreign body obstruction.

Chloride-resistant metabolic alkalosis is uncommonly seen. Chloride-resistant metabolic alkalosis refers to metabolic alkalosis in the setting of a urine chloride concentration of greater than 20 mEq/L. Patients typically have normal or increased ECF volume. These patients, as the name indicates, do not respond to chloride administration. Typically, chloride-resistant metabolic alkalosis is the result of primary hyperaldosteronism, or hyperadrenocorticism. Any condition that increases aldosterone or mineralocorticoid concentration will result in enhanced Na^+ reabsorption and increased excretion of K^+ and H^+ by the kidney, causing alkalosis.

Other causes of metabolic alkalosis include re-feeding syndrome, high dose penicillin, hypoalbuminemia (albumin is a weak acid; see Chapter 11), and post-hypercapnic syndrome.

Diagnosis and clinical signs

Diagnosis of metabolic alkalosis is sometimes overlooked, as it is frequently corrected simply by treatment of the patient's underlying condition. Metabolic alkalosis is characterized by a high pH with a high HCO_3^- (Table 9.1).

Table 9.1 Laboratory characteristics of metabolic alkalosis

Disorder	pH	H+	Primary disturbance	Compensatory response
Metabolic Alkalosis	↑⁻	↓	↑HCO_3^-	↑pCO_2

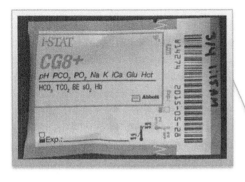
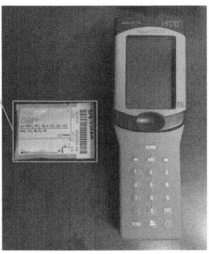

Figure 9.4 Abaxis I-Stat point-of-care blood gas analyzer and a CG8+ cartridge, which is a common device for obtaining quick and reliable blood gas values.

Compensatory increases in pCO_2 may occur. Patients with chloride-responsive metabolic alkalosis have a depletion of extracellular fluid volume (ECFV). A common device used to evaluate electrolyte and acid-base status is the point-of-care Abaxis I-Stat, along with an I-State CG8+ cartridge (Figure 9.4). The CG8+ cartridge includes: Hct, Hgb, iCa, Glu, Na, K, pH, pCO_2, HCO_3^-, TCO_2, BE, pO_2, and SO_2.

The diagnosis of metabolic alkalosis is dependent upon the signs and symptoms of the underlying disease. In humans, metabolic alkalosis may cause neurologic signs that include agitation, disorientation, stupor, and coma. Other clinical signs of metabolic alkalosis include muscle tremors, vomiting, and nausea. A concurrent depletion in potassium is often present, so clinical signs of hypokalemia may occur at the same time. The patient may have weakness, cardiac arrhythmias, or alternations in renal function. Metabolic alkalosis may result in a decrease in ionized calcium, resulting in muscle twitching.

Hypochloremia in metabolic alkalosis will not improve without concurrent supplementation of potassium with chloride, so the addition of potassium chloride to isotonic fluid replacements is indicated for these patients. Low potassium causes hydrogen ions to shift into the cells, causing an increase in extracellular pH. When hypokalemia and hypomagnesemia are both present, the alkalosis will not respond to treatment until the potassium and magnesium deficits are replenished. The administration of other medications may be warranted to treat clinical signs and any underlying conditions. If a mass or a foreign object is suspected to be a cause of GI obstruction, surgery may be required after fluid resuscitation and stabilization.

Metabolic acidosis

Metabolic acidosis is the most common acid-base disturbance seen in small animal practice (DiBartola 2012). According to the traditional approach to acid-base disorders, a patient is likely to have a metabolic acidosis when there is a decrease in HCO_3^-, BE, and pH due to an increase of hydrogen ions. The increase in hydrogen ions is usually caused by a decrease in HCO_3^-, or excess buffering of non-carbonic acid, which results in acidemia (DiBartola 2012). The respiratory system compensates by increased ventilation and subsequent decrease in pCO_2. The etiology of the metabolic acidosis may be determined by considering the anion gap and chloride levels, loss of HCO_3^-, or gain of H^+ (Norkus 2012).

Pathophysiology

There are four primary processes through which metabolic acidosis can occur. These processes include loss of HCO_3^-, increased acid production, inability to excrete H^+, or addition of exogenous acids to the body. The clinical appearance of the patient will be determined largely by the underlying disorder.

Loss of HCO_3^- rich fluids may result from small bowel diarrhea. Increased acid production is a result of increased cellular metabolism that causes an increase in formation of byproducts, including lactic acid, CO_2 and H^+. Causes of increased cellular metabolism include excessive exercise, seizures, and hypovolemic shock. The excess H^+ is buffered by HCO_3^-, resulting in hypobicarbonatemia. This results in a low HCO_3^- to pCO_2 ratio. The respiratory system compensates through hyperventilation, allowing the patient to blow off excess CO_2 This effectively lowers the pCO_2, and rapidly minimizes changes in pH. Metabolic acidosis with a normal anion gap is seen when there is a decrease in HCO_3^- with an increase in Cl^-, which maintains the anion gap within normal limits (Norkus 2012). An elevated anion gap with a decrease in HCO_3^- is indicative of a normochloremic metabolic acidosis. In these cases, the Cl^- levels are not affected.

Renal system dysfunction can result in metabolic acidosis in several ways. The kidney's primary job is to excrete waste along with H^+ and ammonia. In acute or chronic kidney disease, metabolic acidosis results from glomerular malfunction where one or both may not be excreted normally, resulting in buildup in the bloodstream. Urine specific gravity, blood urea nitrogen, creatinine, and phosphate levels should all be evaluated in conjunction with acid-base balance

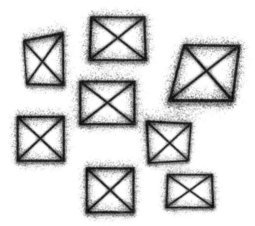

Figure 9.5 Calcium oxalate crystals form as a result of glycolic acid formation from ingesting ethylene glycol.

to assess renal function. When abnormalities occur, acute kidney injury or chronic kidney disease should be considered in evaluation and stabilization of the patient.

Increase production of acids can occur in patients with diabetic ketoacidosis due to production of excess ketones, or production of lactic acidosis such as in patients with heatstroke or shock. A common example of the addition of exogenous acid resulting in metabolic acidosis is the ingestion of ethylene glycol. Ethylene glycol is the primary ingredient in most radiator fluid products. Animals are attracted to ethylene glycol because of its sweet taste. Although ethylene glycol is not toxic, it is metabolized into toxic products in the liver. Toxic metabolites of ethylene glycol cause an osmolar gap that transitions to an increased anion gap metabolic acidosis. See Figure 9.5.

Diagnosis and clinical signs

Recognition of metabolic acidosis is critical for veterinary medical staff, as quick recognition leads to prompt response and treatment of the patient. If left untreated, metabolic acidosis can result in many detrimental effects, including shock and/or death. Familiarity with clinical signs and knowledge of the effects of metabolic acidosis on pH, pCO_2, HCO_3^-, BE, and the anion gap are essential when assisting a veterinarian who may be treating a patient with an acid-base disorder. A low pH (indicating elevated $[H^+]$) with decreased bicarbonate levels characterizes metabolic acidosis. pH derangement should be suspected in any patient with a disease process that may be associated with acidosis, i.e. ketoacidosis or acute kidney injury. An acid-base assessment should be performed on these patients to confirm and monitor for resolution throughout treatment.

Table 9.2 Laboratory characteristics of metabolic acidosis

Disorder	pH	H⁺	Primary disturbance	Compensatory response
Metabolic Acidosis	↓	↑	$\downarrow HCO_3^-$	$\downarrow pCO_2$

Clinical signs of metabolic acidosis vary, and are largely dependent on their underlying disease (Table 9.2). Several common clinical signs may be present in patients with metabolic acidosis, including tachypnea, nausea, vomiting, and malaise. Hyperpnea, or Kussmaul respiration, may also be noted and is a characteristic sign that consists of long deep breaths at a normal respiratory rate, indicating a compensatory effort to increase ventilation. The key to accurate diagnosis is a thorough evaluation that includes a complete medical history and laboratory analysis. A patient suffering from metabolic acidosis may exhibit diarrhea, fever, lethargy, and/or tachypnea (hyperventilation). The acidosis itself has many deleterious effects that include decreased cardiac output, decreased blood pressure, decreased hepatic and renal perfusion, decreased myocardial contractility (predisposing the patient to cardiac arrhythmias), arterial dilation, and insulin resistance. Patients with metabolic acidosis are frequently tachypneic and may exhibit Kussmaul respiration as the disorder progresses. These changes are due to compensatory efforts by the respiratory system to increase ventilation and exchange of CO_2.

Treatment of metabolic acidosis

Treatment of metabolic acidosis includes addressing the underlying cause of the metabolic acidosis. In most cases, treatment of the underlying disorder will allow resolution of acidosis without administration of sodium bicarbonate (Figure 9.6). Administration of activated charcoal in the cases of toxicity due to ingestion is typically warranted in an effort to reduce absorption of the toxin through the gastrointestinal tract. Diuretics may be utilized in certain cases. Supplementation with electrolytes is required in most patients but especially during the administration of diuretics, as well as for many other disease processes. In patients undergoing diuresis, care must be taken to prevent fluid overload, especially in patients with an underlying heart condition. As in metabolic alkalosis, correction of electrolyte abnormalities is also key in correcting this acid-base derangement. Judicious supplementation with sodium bicarbonate ($NaHCO_3^-$) may be indicated in certain patients when the body buffer is not sufficient for the amount of H⁺ present in the body. If the patient's pH is less than 7.1–7.2 with an HCO_3^- (or TCO_2) less than 10 mmol/L, sodium bicarbonate therapy may be indicated. Only enough $NaHCO_3^-$ to raise the pH to, or just above, 7.2 should be given (Mazzaferro 2013). Recommended calculations for bicarbonate supplementation vary, but the following is often used:

$$0.4 \times \text{bodyweight (kg)} \times \text{base deficit}$$

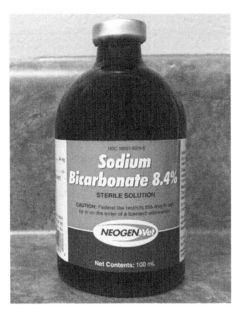

Figure 9.6 Image of an 8.4% sodium bicarbonate ($NaHCO_3^-$) injectable solution bottle.

Half of the calculated amount should be administered IV slowly. Alternatively some use a standard replacement of 0.5–1 mEq per kg bodyweight. The half dose should be given once, preferably over 4–6 hr. Check bicarbonate and pH levels within 2 hr after the half dose has been completed. If the bicarbonate level is up to 12, or the pH is up to 7.2, do not repeat the other half of the dose. Caution must be taken with giving bicarbonate as rapid administration can result in coronary acidosis, causing a sudden death. Also if the patient is severely obtunded and unable to regulate ventilation to compensate for the increased pCO_2 that results from the metabolism of exogenous bicarbonate, a paradoxical cerebro-spinal fluid acidosis may occur that can cause rapid death. Other complications that occur from $NaHCO_3^-$ administration include hypernatremia, hypokalemia, hypocalcemia, iatrogenic metabolic alkalosis, or volume overload due to the large amount of sodium administered with the bicarbonate. Therefore, use of sodium bicarbonate must be weighed against the potential risks to the patient and administered judiciously.

Prognosis of metabolic acid-base derangements

Early detection and treatment of any acid-base derangement is key. Since the respiratory system responds to metabolic derangements quickly, metabolic blood gas disorders are usually diagnosed once the compensatory response systems have already kicked in. If the underlying disease, as well as primary disturbance, is promptly and properly treated, the compensatory response and any other clinical signs should resolve accordingly. Prognosis varies and is ultimately dependent on the underlying cause and concurrent diseases present. Treating electrolyte abnormalities in conjunction with the acid-base disturbance and understanding compensatory mechanisms is a critical skill for diagnosis and treatment of any metabolic acid-base disorders. Technicians having a solid understanding of these disorders are invaluable to the veterinarian and will aid in the early detection and diagnosis of a metabolic blood gas disorder in our patients.

References

Battaglia, A. (ed.), (2007). *Small Animal Emergency and Critical Care for Veterinary Technicians*, 2nd ed. St Louis, MO: Saunders Elsevier: 15–19.

Bryant, S. (ed.). (2013). *Anesthesia for Veterinary Technicians*. New York: John Wiley & Sons: 91–3.

de Morais, H. A. & DiBartola, S. (eds), (2008). *Veterinary Clinics of North America Small Animal Practice: Advances in fluid, electrolyte and acid-base disorders*: **38**(3): 435–47. Philadelphia: Elsevier Saunders.

DiBartola, S. (ed.), (2012). *Fluid, Electrolyte, and Acid-Base Disorders in Small Animal Practice*, 4th ed. St Louis, MO: Elsevier Saunders. 231–86.

Irizarry, R. & Reiss, A. (2009). Arterial and venous blood gases: Indications, interpretations, and clinical applications. *Compendium: Continuing Education for Veterinarians* **31**: 1–7.

Mazzaferro, E. (2013). *Small Animal Fluid, Electrolyte and Acid-Base Disorders: A Color Handbook*. London: Manson Publishing.

Norkus, C. (ed.). (2012). *Veterinary Technician's Manual for Small Animal Emergency and Critical Care*. Chichester: Wiley-Blackwell.

Reece, W. (2009). *Functional Anatomy and Physiology of Domestic Animals*, 4th ed. Ames, IA: Wiley-Blackwell.

Thomas, J. A. & Lerche, P. (2011). *Anesthesia and Analgesia for Veterinary Technicians*. St Louis, MO: Elsevier Mosby.

Waddell, L. (2013). The practitioner's acid-base primer obtaining and interpreting blood gases. *Today's Veterinary Practice*: 43–4, http://todaysveterinarypractice.navc.com/the-practitioners-acid-base-primer-obtaining-interpreting-blood-gases/.

CHAPTER 10

Respiratory Acid-Base Disorders

Paula Plummer, LVT, VTS (ECC, SAIM)

Evaluating a patient's ability to effectively oxygenate and ventilate involves a complete physical examination and diagnostic testing. Blood gases can assist greatly in assessing the functionality of the respiratory system, including gas exchange. Respiratory acid-base abnormalities are determined by alterations of the partial pressure of arterial carbon dioxide ($PaCO_2$), indicating changes in ventilation, which in turn cause alterations in the pH. The partial pressure of arterial oxygen (PaO_2) denotes the oxygenation status of that individual. This chapter will cover respiratory acid-base abnormalities, including respiratory acidosis, respiratory alkalosis, and disorders of oxygenation.

The respiratory system

The drive to breathe comes from the respiratory center located in the medulla of the brain. An entire matrix is devoted to making the body breathe. Respiratory rate, pattern, and the generation of a breath is controlled by the respiratory center. The pons, cerebellum, and forebrain are responsible for breathing but are not required for one to be able to breath. This occurs due to chemoreceptors and chemoreflexes that feed the respiratory center with information about carbon dioxide and oxygen levels within the body. A negative feedback system designed to detect alterations in alveolar ventilation will detect changes to pH, carbon dioxide, and oxygen levels. Chemoreceptors are located in the peripheral and central nervous system to keep alveolar ventilation regulated. The ventilatory control system is governed by a series of mechanoreflexes throughout the chest wall as well as pulmonary and airway receptors. These receptors detect changes in pressure, temperature, and stretch. Depending on the location, the receptor will notice change and cause the body to correct itself, i.e. cough, bronchoconstriction,

Acid-Base and Electrolyte Handbook for Veterinary Technicians, First Edition.
Edited by Angela Randels-Thorp and David Liss.
© 2017 John Wiley & Sons, Inc. Published 2017 by John Wiley & Sons, Inc.
Companion website: www.wiley.com/go/liss/electrolytes

or change respiratory rate. This control system will help regulate blood gas hemostasis (Johnson & de Morais 2012).

The respiratory system functions include oxygenation and elimination of carbon dioxide. The lungs are only attached to the thoracic cavity near the mediastinum. The lungs are kept lubricated during movement by pleural fluid, which is a thin layer of fluid that surrounds the lungs (Hall 2011a). A normal small amount of suction is present in the thoracic cavity; it is also known as pleural pressure. Pleural pressure that is present in the pleura creates a negative pressure. As inspiration occurs, the negative pressure increases, drawing a breath in; when the negative pressure is decreased during expiration, the breath is released from the lungs.

Contraction and relaxation of the diaphragm along with the respiratory muscles and the negative pressure within the pleural cavity are all required for normal respiration. Inspiration occurs when the diaphragm contracts, the ribs move forward and outward, and respiratory muscles relax in order to enlarge the thoracic cavity. When the abdominal muscles relax the abdominal organs will move caudally to allow for enlargement of the pleural cavity as the diaphragm contracts. As the thoracic cavity enlarges the air will be taken in through the nostrils, down into the lungs via the bronchial tree, and finally to the alveoli (Heath & Atkins 2012; Hall 2011a). Expiration occurs as the abdominal muscles contract, pushing the abdominal organs back to their normal position. This causes the diaphragm to return to its normal position, pushing the air out of the respiratory system. The thoracic cavity will then return to its normal size during expiration.

Once the air is in the lungs, a process known as diffusion will carry the oxygen from the alveoli to the pulmonary circulation then throughout the body (Figure 10.1). Carbon dioxide is diffused from circulation in the lungs and

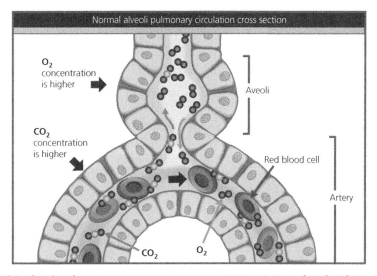

Figure 10.1 Alveoli pulmonary cross-section. (Source: VIN 2014. Reproduced with permission of Veterinary Information Network, Inc.)

expelled from the body. Diffusion is the motion of molecules across a membrane from an area of higher concentration to an area of lower concentration. All gases in respiratory physiology are free to move among fluids and tissues within the body. An energy source will provide kinetic energy to allow the molecules to rapidly move in any direction. The movement of a molecule from a highly con-centrated area to a low-concentrated area to equalize the concentration keeps oxygen and carbon dioxide at normal levels.

The partial pressure of a gas is the amount of pressure caused by the impact of the molecule on the surface of the gas. The amount of pressure that is applied to the surface is directly related to the amount of gas molecules present (Hall 2011b). Oxygen is absorbed from the alveoli into pulmonary circulation, and new oxygen is inspired continuously. When oxygen is absorbed faster, the alve-oli concentration will decrease, and the higher the respiratory rate, the higher the oxygen concentration becomes. Alveolar oxygen concentration and alveolar partial pressure of oxygen (PaO_2) is dependent on the rate of absorption of oxygen into circulation and how fast new oxygen is entered into the body (res-piratory rate). The alveolar partial pressure of carbon dioxide ($PaCO_2$) will be determined by alveolar ventilation. The level of $PaCO_2$ will be increased with a lower rate of excretion of carbon dioxide and increased with a higher rate of excretion of carbon dioxide. When the respiratory rate or tidal volume decreases, $PaCO_2$ levels will increase.

Oxygen

Oxygen delivery is the body's ability to transport the oxygen from the alveoli to body tissue. Oxygen is carried to the tissue in two forms: dissolved or bound to hemoglobin. Hemoglobin is the primary carrier of oxygen. Each hemoglobin molecule is capable of carrying four oxygen molecules. Under normal respira-tory function the oxygen will bind to all four receptors, causing an oxygen saturation of greater than 97%. Once the oxygen is bound to the hemoglobin, it is transported to tissue via circulation. The oxygen capacity can be determined by the amount of oxygen that can be combined with hemoglobin and can be determined by the oxygen hemoglobin dissociation curve.

When looking at the oxygen hemoglobin disassociation curve (Figure 10.2), the amount of hemoglobin that is bound to oxygen will increase with an increase in PaO_2. Notice in Figure 10.2 that the higher the PaO_2 rises the curve flattens out and only a small amount of hemoglobin is added at the top of the curve.

Several conditions can alter hemoglobin-binding characteristics with oxygen molecules. When these are present, the curve will shift to the right or left, depend-ing on the dysfunction. Conditions that cause a right shift include respiratory acidosis, increased $PaCO_2$, hyperthermia, and increased 2,3 diphosphoglycerate (2,3 DPG). The right shift causes oxygen to separate from hemoglobin, delivering more oxygen to tissue (Hall 2011c). 2,3 DPG is an organophosphate that binds to hemoglobin like oxygen.

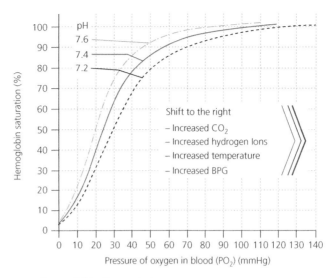

Figure 10.2 Oxygen hemoglobin disassociation curve.

A shift to the left in the curve is caused by the reverse of conditions that cause a right shift and acute respiratory alkalemia. Please see acute respiratory alkalosis in the "Respiratory alkalosis" section for etiologies. The affinity of hemoglobin oxygen is increased, which will reduce the amount of oxygen that is released to the tissue. Chronic respiratory alkalemia will cause an increase in 2,3 DPG; therefore, the oxygen hemoglobin disassociation curve will return to normal (Johnson & de Morais 2012). Once $PaCO_2$ levels and hydrogen levels are decreased, the oxygen hemoglobin disassociation curve will shift to the left (Hall 2011d).

Carbon dioxide

Carbon dioxide plays an important role in acid-base regulation. Carbon dioxide excess is converted into bicarbonate and released into the plasma. Carbonic acid is formed and then quickly separates to hydrogen and bicarbonate intracellularly. Hemostasis is kept by hydrogen (H^+) and chloride (Cl^-) diffusing from plasma to erythrocytes and vice versa. This process is termed the chloride shift (Johnson & de Morais 2012). Exhalation through the lungs is the primary mechanism of carbon dioxide excretion. However, the kidneys play a small role in excretion of carbon dioxide. The elimination of carbon dioxide from the body is important to prevent respiratory acidosis.

Respiratory acidosis

Respiratory acidosis is an acid-base disturbance that is demonstrated by an increase in $PaCO_2$. It is also termed hypercapnia and indicated alveolar hypoventilation. Alveolar ventilation is maintained by tidal volume and respiratory rate. When the respiratory rate or tidal volume decreases, carbon dioxide will be retained and the level of $PaCO_2$ increases (greater than 45 mmHg), leading to a decrease in pH (less than 7.35) and causing a respiratory acidosis. The body will naturally compensate by increasing bicarbonate levels, although this is not an acute compensatory mechanism. Simply stated, respiratory acidosis will occur when elimination of carbon dioxide via the respiratory system cannot keep up with the production amount of carbon dioxide (Johnson & de Morais 2012).

Both acute and chronic respiratory acidosis can occur. Determining whether the respiratory acidosis is either chronic or acute will help determine the etiology of the acid-base disorder. Diagnosis of the acute or chronic phase of acidosis can be done by determining whether the amount of compensation is typical or atypical.

An acute increase in $PaCO_2$ will cause the carbon dioxide intracellularly to naturally increase. An increase in carbon dioxide causes intracellular (hemoglobin) and extracellular (plasma protein) buffers to return carbon dioxide levels to normal. In acute respiratory acidosis, every 1 mmHg increase in $PaCO_2$ will cause a compensation of an increase in bicarbonate at a rate of 0.15 mEq/L in dogs and cats (Johnson & de Morais 2012). The initial phase of compensation for a respiratory acid-base derangement begins immediately with changes of bicarbonate due to titration of intracellular non-bicarbonate buffers. Within hours the kidneys will start to reabsorb the bicarbonate and alter acid excretion to return the derangement to normal (DiBartola 2012).

If respiratory acidosis persists, maximal renal compensation will occur within 2–5 days. Hydrogen concentrations will become increased in the renal tubular cells with chronic respiratory acidosis. As a result bicarbonate is reabsorbed and chloride is excreted through the urine. Chloruresis and hypochloremia are the result. A new "normal" is reached within the body when increased plasma bicarbonate is equal to the increased renal reabsorption of bicarbonate. In chronic respiratory acidosis, every 1 mmHg increase in $PaCO_2$ will cause a compensation of an increase in bicarbonate at a rate of 0.35 mEq/L in dogs. Compensation values in chronic respiratory acidosis are not known in cats (Johnson and & de Morais 2012).

Etiologies of chronic respiratory acidosis include pathology in which alveolar ventilation, respiratory drive, or functionality of the respiratory system is impaired or increased dead space occurs (Johnson & de Morais 2012; Monning 2013).

There are many risk factors for respiratory acidosis. They include the following upper-airway diseases that include aspiration pneumonitis, neoplasia, tracheal collapse, laryngeal diseases, or an obstructed endotracheal tube. An impaired respiratory center can cause respiratory acidosis. Neurologic diseases that include brainstem or spinal cord lesions as well as drug-induced respiratory depression, such as neuromuscular blocking agents, are included in this group of risk factors. Classes of pharmacologic agents that can contribute to respiratory acidosis include general anesthetic agents, inhalants, opioids, tranquilizers, sedatives, and hypnotics. These agents will depress the respiratory center, decrease the respiratory drive, and in return cause carbon dioxide to build up (McDonnel & Kerr 2007). Events such as cardiopulmonary arrest, heatstroke, or hyperthermia can increase carbon dioxide production and decrease alveolar ventilation, causing respiratory acidosis. Pulmonary and lower airway diseases such as acute respiratory distress syndrome (ARDS), chronic obstructive pulmonary disease (COPD), asthma, pulmonary edema, pulmonary embolism (PE), pneumonia, fibrosis, metastatic disease, and smoke inhalation can lead to respiratory acidosis. Extra pulmonary causes for respiratory acidosis usually fall under trauma and can include incidents such as diaphragmatic hernia, pneumothorax, and pleural space disorders or flail chest (Hall 2011d). And finally inappropriate mechanical ventilation and profound obesity in a patient are risk factors for respiratory acidosis (Monning 2013).

Clinical signs seen in respiratory acidosis are specific to the underlying disease process. If the patient is diagnosed with chronic respiratory acidosis, they will show mild clinical signs or be asymptomatic. Other non-specific clinical signs of respiratory acidosis can include cardiovascular, metabolic, or neurologic clinical signs. Tachyarrhythmia is seen as a result of stimulation of the sympathetic nervous system releasing catecholamines and will cause an increased heart rate, cardiac output, decrease contractility, and systemic vascular resistance. Because of this on physical examination tachycardia, hypertension, and red mucous membranes are present. It is typical for the severity of clinical signs to be increased in a patient experiencing acute respiratory acidosis versus a patient in a chronic disease state (DiBartola 2012; Monning 2013). However, if a patient with chronic respiratory acidosis decompensates, life-threatening clinical signs can arise and should be treated immediately.

It is common for hypercapnic patients to be concurrently hypoxic. Patients go into cardiopulmonary arrest from hypoxemia faster than from hypercapnia. It is beneficial for most patients to receive oxygen therapy during an acute respiratory acidosis event (de Morais & DiBartola 2009). As mentioned above in the "Oxygen" section of this chapter, acute respiratory acidosis will cause a right shift to the oxygen hemoglobin disassociation curve. The right shift will cause an increase of the oxygen level in the tissue and increase oxygen-carrying capacity and delivery.

An arterial blood gas is the diagnostic test of choice for a definitive diagnosis of a respiratory acid-base disorder. A quick diagnosis of respiratory acidosis and aggressive treatment of the underlying condition causing the acid-base disorder is the best treatment plan. Providing the patient with proper alveolar ventilation and oxygenation is the ultimate outcome in a patient experiencing acute respiratory acidosis. Elimination of the underlying condition, i.e. upper-airway foreign body removal or discontinuation of medications or performing a thoracocentesis to remove air or fluid from the thoracic cavity, should be performed in a timely manner. Patients experiencing respiratory muscle fatigue or respiratory failure may need to be mechanically ventilated. Positive pressure ventilation is indicated in patients with a $PaCO_2$ of 60 mmHg or greater and is hypoxemic (PaO_2 of less than 60 mmHg) in the face of oxygen therapy (Haskins 2007).

Treatment with sodium bicarbonate ($NaHCO_3$) is contraindicated in the patient with respiratory acidosis. $NaHCO_3$ administration will alter the respiratory drive, making hypoxemia worse with an increased $PaCO_2$ and in return worsening respiratory failure (Johnson & de Morais 2006). $NaHCO_3$ administration can also cause hypotension, decrease cardiac contractility, decrease blood flow to the brain, and even cause cardiac arrest. In most patients, the risk of $NaHCO_3$ outweighs the benefits and it is not the treatment of choice.

If the arterial blood gas shows chronic respiratory acidosis, oxygen therapy should be used with caution. Normally carbon dioxide is what drives the respiratory center; therefore, when the carbon dioxide is increased, respiration will be triggered. When a patient is in a state of chronic respiratory acidosis, the level of carbon dioxide in the body is always higher than normal and carbon dioxide receptors become depressed. Because of this, the patient stays in a normal state of hypoxia and hypercapnia. The respiratory center will not be triggered to take a breath until the PaO_2 is less than 60 mmHg. Therefore, if patient is given supplemental oxygen their depressed respiratory carbon dioxide receptors will not trigger respiration when PaO_2 is above 60 mmHg (Randels 2013).

Respiratory alkalosis

Respiratory alkalosis is an increase in the body's pH (greater than 7.45) and a decrease in $PaCO_2$ (less than 35 mmHg), also known as hypocapnia. The body will naturally compensate by increasing bicarbonate levels. Respiratory alkalosis can be acute or chronic just as in respiratory acidosis.

In acute respiratory alkalosis the $PaCO_2$ has been decreased rapidly making the body find a new "normal." Chloride becomes extracellular, making bicarbonate become intracellular, causing decreased plasma bicarbonate levels. Plasma proteins and intracellular phosphate are the buffers in the compensation process. In acute respiratory alkalosis every 1 mmHg decrease of $PaCO_2$ will cause a compensatory decrease of 0.25 mEq/L in bicarbonate in dogs and cats (Johnson & de Morais 2012).

During chronic respiratory alkalosis, the body has had time to appropriately compensate by normalizing pH. Every 1 mmHg decrease in $PaCO_2$ will cause a compensatory response of 0.55 mEq/L decrease of bicarbonate. Patients experiencing chronic respiratory alkalosis will have varying degrees of abnormal $PaCO_2$ and bicarbonate with a normal pH due to the compensation process taking up to four weeks. Just because patients exhibit these results on their blood gas results does not indicate a mixed acid-base disorder (DiBartola 2012). Mixed acid-base disorders are reviewed in detail in a separate chapter of this textbook.

Various conditions potentially causing respiratory alkalosis include hypoxemia, primary pulmonary disease, processes activating the respiratory center, inappropriate mechanical ventilation, or external stimulation that resulted in pain or anxiety (Johnson & de Morais 2006). Pulmonary diseases such as pneumonia, PTE, pulmonary edema, and ARDS can cause respiratory alkalosis. Activation of the central respiratory center causes respiratory alkalosis. Liver disease, hyperadrenocorticism, gram-negative sepsis, drugs (salicylates, corticosteroids, progesterone, and xanthine-aminophylline), over compensation of respiratory acidosis, central neurologic disease, exercise, and heatstroke will cause activation of the central respiratory center. Classes of pharmaceutical drugs such as salicylates, corticosteroids, progesterone, and xanthine can all be a contributing cause of respiratory alkalosis. Salicylates include aspirin, sodium salicylate, and bismuth among others. This class of drugs is typically used to treat inflammation. At toxic doses, they will directly affect the respiratory center, causing hyperventilation and then depression (Boothe 2011). Overcompensation of respiratory acidosis will result in respiratory alkalosis. Central neurologic diseases that can result in respiratory alkalosis include trauma, neoplasia, infection, and inflammation.

As with respiratory acidosis, clinical signs of respiratory alkalosis are not specific to the acid-base disturbance. The clinical signs will be specific to the underlying condition. With an increased pH of 7.6 or above, vasoconstriction, metabolic, cardiopulmonary, or neurologic dysfunction may occur. Hypocapnia that results in a $PaCO_2$ of less than 25 mmHg will decrease cerebral blood flow, potentially causing seizures or altered mentation (Johnson & de Morais 2006). A direct treatment for respiratory alkalosis is not available. However, treatment of the underlying condition will correct respiratory alkalosis.

Patients that have existing cardiac disease can exhibit supraventricular and ventricular arrhythmias due to the positive ionotropic effect of alkalosis on the heart. Patients that are experiencing acute respiratory alkalosis will have a left shift in the oxygen hemoglobin disassociation curve, as mentioned earlier in the "Oxygen" section of this chapter. The left shift will decrease the rate of oxygen release to the tissue. If the state of respiratory alkalosis progresses to a chronic condition, the left shift will return to normal because erythrocytes will increase production of 2,3 DPG, therefore returning the oxygen hemoglobin disassociation curve to normal (Johnson & de Morais 2012).

Disorders of oxygenation

Hypoxia is the lack of oxygen in the tissue and hypoxemia is the lack of oxygen in blood. These two terms are often used interchangeably but actually have different definitions. As stated previously, PaO_2 is the partial pressure of the arterial oxygen and PAO_2 is the partial pressure of the alveolar oxygen content.

Etiologies of hypoxemia include a diffusion impairment, hypoventilation, V/Q mismatch, or right to left shunt. PaO_2 is the value that is necessary to assess the oxygenation status of the patient on an arterial blood gas sample. Fraction of inspired oxygen (FiO_2) is the concentration of oxygen the patient is inspiring. Room air is considered an FiO_2 of 21% or 0.21. A normal PaO_2 is considered 4–5 times the amount of FiO_2. Therefore, the normal PaO_2 of a patient breathing room air is 80–100 mmHg or the normal PaO_2 of a patient breathing 100% oxygen is 400–500 mmHg. The oxygenation of a patient cannot be assessed on a venous blood sample. Venous blood samples have already had the oxygen consumed from them. Therefore, venous blood will not properly assess oxygenation (Haskins 2004).

If the capability of obtaining an arterial blood sample to assess the oxygenation of the patient is not available, the pulse oximeter and oxygen hemoglobin disassociation curve can be used to help determine oxygen saturation of the patient. The pulse oximeter is a common monitoring device used in veterinary medicine to help determine saturation of hemoglobin with oxygen and can assist in evaluating oxygenation. It is important to know that the pulse oximeter determines the percentage of hemoglobin that is saturated with oxygen by an LED infrared wavelength. The oxygen hemoglobin disassociation curve can be used as an aide with pulse oximetry to determine the oxygenation status of the patient. The oxygen hemoglobin disassociation curve shows when the hemoglobin saturation is at 92% the PaO_2 is 80 mmHg. It is recommended that when the PaO_2 is less than 70 mmHg or were hemoglobin saturation is 90%, oxygen therapy should be initiated (Tseng & Drobatz 2004).

Clinical signs of the hypoxic patient include cyanosis, dyspnea, panting, tachypnea, tachycardia, or open mouth breathing. The body position of the dyspneic patient can be an indicator as well. If the canine patient will not rest, stands consistently, abducts elbows, or extends their neck, this will be an indicator of dyspnea. The feline patient will lie sternally but not touch the floor and while in this position they can subtly abduct their elbows. Another body position the feline patient displays will be neck extension but in a less obvious manner than their canine counterpart.

Providing supplemental oxygen for the hypoxic patient is the initial therapy of choice. Supplemental oxygen can be provided in several different ways: oxygen cage, intranasal catheter(s), face mask, nasal prongs, or oxygen hood are common methods used in veterinary medicine. The feline patient will be most tolerable of an oxygen cage or the oxygen hood. With the canine patient breed, underlying condition and toleration of the therapy method should be taken into consideration. Patients that are at risk for increased intracranial pressure should not receive oxygen via intranasal catheters or prongs, because of the risk of sneezing, which will lead to an even further increase in intracranial pressure. Some canine patients will paw at or remove the intranasal catheter or prongs due to irritation. Then the method of which they are receiving oxygen must be altered. Figure 10.3 and Figure 10.4 are examples of oxygen supplementation techniques that can be used to provide oxygen therapy to patients.

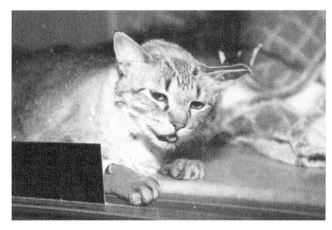

Figure 10.3 Dyspneic cat.

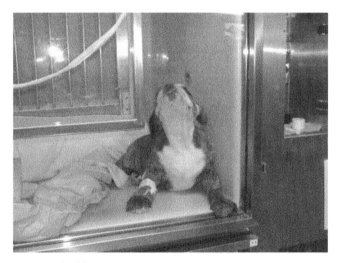

Figure 10.4 Respiratory bulldog.

Whatever method of oxygen administration is chosen, it should be humidified. Humidification will keep the patient's mucous membranes and mucous secretions moist and this will help prevent infection and irritation in the respiratory tract (Tseng & Drobatz 2004).

Placement of the intranasal cannula can be done unilaterally or bilaterally. A numbing agent, such as proparacaine, is placed in the nostril. A red rubber catheter is measured from the medial canthus of the eye to the end of the nares and marked at that point. It is inserted intranasally to the mark and secured with either skin glue or suture placement. The oxygen flow rate for each cannula should not exceed 100 ml/kg or 4 L/min. At this rate the oxygen concentration is estimated to be 40% (Crowe 2009). If rates of oxygen flow exceed the recommended rate, it can cause irritation or drying of the mucous membranes. See Figure 10.5.

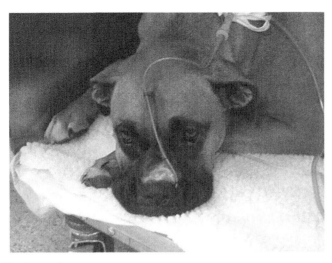

Figure 10.5 Nasal cannula.

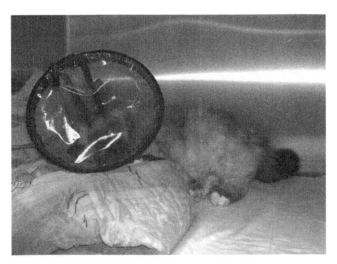

Figure 10.6 Dyspneic cat with oxygen hood.

An oxygen cage can be adapted from an incubator, small cage, or induction chamber if a commercial oxygen cage is not available. Temperature control, oxygen level, and humidity in the cage are important to monitor when adapting a cage into an oxygen cage. Commercial oxygen monitor, thermometers, and in-line humidifiers can be purchased to place in the cages. A commercial oxygen cage can administer 21–60%, depending on the cage's abilities.

The oxygen hood can be bought commercially or an Elizabethan collar can be adapted into an oxygen hood (Figure 10.6). If adapting an Elizabethan collar, only cover two-thirds of the front surface with clear plastic wrap to help with temperature control of the patient. A humidified oxygen line can be secured

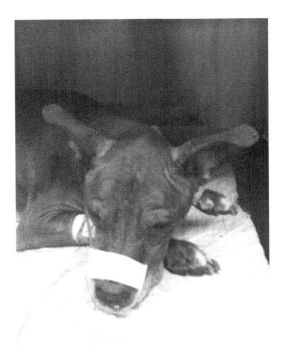

Figure 10.7 Nasal prongs.

inside the back of the Elizabethan collar as an oxygen source. An oxygen concentration of up to 80% can be obtained with this method of oxygen therapy. Monitoring the percentage of oxygen in the hood can be challenging. In lieu of monitoring the oxygen percentage, monitoring the patient for clinical signs of dyspnea can be done (Crowe 2009).

Nasal prongs are a cheap and convenient method to administer oxygen therapy (Figure 10.7). The prongs are placed in the patient's nares and secured in place by skin glue or suture placement. An Elizabethan collar is helpful to prevent the patient from removing the device. The oxygen flow rate should not exceed 100 ml/kg or 4 L/min. At this rate the oxygen concentration is estimated to be 40% (Crowe 2009). If rates of oxygen flow exceed the recommended rate, it can cause irritation or drying of the mucous membranes.

There are pros and cons to each method of oxygen supplementation. It is important to use the best method for the patient and your clinic. See Table 10.1 for the pros and cons of each oxygen therapy administration technique.

Complications from oxygen therapy such as oxygen toxicity, hypercarbia, and atelectasis can occur. If 100% oxygen is administered for longer than 24–72 hr, patients can be at risk of a complication called oxygen toxicity. Clinical signs include: pulmonary edema, pleural effusion, and changes to the airway epithelium. The least amount of oxygen supplementation required to adequately

Table 10.1 Pros and cons of oxygen therapy techniques

Method	Pros	Cons
Face mask	Simple Inexpensive Convenient Fairly effective Anesthesia machine can be used instead of wall oxygen	Most patients will not tolerate mask on face Can be stressful to patient Requires individual attention to ensure patient is receiving oxygen
Nasal prongs	Convenient Inexpensive Effective on recumbent patients Secured with skin staples	Unless patient is recumbent they can be dislodged from patient easily Exact FiO_2 unknown
Nasal cannulas	Secured easily with skin staples Unilateral/bilateral Easy patient monitoring	Discomfort and constant irritation for patient Elizabethan collar is needed so patient doesn't remove cannulas Potential patient sedation for placement
Oxygen cage	Convenient Temperature controlled Exact FiO_2 known Less stress for patient Provides quiet environment for patient	Expense Requires hands off patient monitoring FiO_2 drops when door is opened Cage maintenance Size limitation of patient Overheating of patients
Oxygen hood	Convenient Inexpensive Used on large patients Patients tolerate this method more than they do nasal cannulas	Hard to manage unless patient is recumbent Exact FiO_2 unknown Patient can overheat

oxygenate the patient should be used. For long-term use, supplementation should be less than 50% (Tseng & Drobatz 2004).

Hypoventilation

Hypoventilation is diagnosed in a patient when $PaCO_2$ is greater than 40 mmHg and is caused by a decrease in alveolar ventilation (Heath & Atkins 2012; Hackett 2009). The arterial oxygen content is equalized by the balance of removal of oxygen from the body and the body being replenished with oxygen by arterial ventilation. If alveolar ventilation decreases, this results in a decrease in arterial and alveolar oxygen levels (hypoxemia) and an increase of arterial and alveolar carbon dioxide levels (hypercapnia) When supplemental oxygen is administered it will decrease the $PaCO_2$, correcting hypoventilation.

Etiologies for hypoventilation include primary lung disease, V/Q mismatch, right to left shunt, respiratory center depression (due to anesthesia), central nervous system dysfunction, or disease affecting the functionality of the respiratory tract.

Diffusion impairment

Diffusion impairment causes hypoxemia by not allowing normal diffusion between oxygen and capillary blood in the alveoli. The oxygen concentration, surface area, and thickness of the membrane will determine the capability of oxygen diffusion. Diseases that cause thickening of the membrane or decrease of surface area will slow diffusion, causing hypoxemia. Treatment for diffusion impairment is to supplement oxygen. Patients that are experiencing hypoxemia due to diffusion impairment will respond to oxygen supplementation (Hackett 2009). See "Disorders of oxygenation" section for supplemental choices and therapies.

V/Q mismatch

V/Q mismatch occurs when blood flow (perfusion) does not closely correlate with gas exchange (ventilation) (Hackett 2009). Pulmonary perfusion is controlled locally and a decrease in oxygen level in the alveoli will cause vasoconstriction of the blood vessels to ensure the blood is distributed properly. Local hypoperfusion in the lungs can occur because of narrowing of the airway, fluid accumulation in the parenchyma, or edema. Due to the underlying condition, the localized area is not able to ventilate correctly, causing the oxygen level to decrease and the carbon dioxide level to increase, causing a V/Q mismatch. This type of V/Q mismatch is typically responsive to oxygen therapy (Haskins 2004). Causes of low V/Q mismatch (poor ventilation and efficiently perfused), of less than 0.1, include pulmonary diseases such as: pneumonia, pulmonary edema, and atelectasis. A patient experiencing atelectasis or alveolar collapse can be positionally rotated or have the portion of collapsed lung opened with positive pressure ventilation. Until the underlying condition is corrected, the V/Q mismatch in these situations will not be corrected (Haskins 2004).

A high V/Q mismatch (poor perfusion and efficiently ventilated) is greater than 1. A high V/Q mismatch is typically found with underlying conditions such as emphysema or pulmonary thromboembolism (Haskins 2006; Hackett 2009).

V/Q mismatch is the most common etiology of hypoxemia (Balakrishnan & King 2014). The Alveolar-arterial gradient can be used to assess the respiratory function, and identify the presence and severity of a V/Q mismatch (Johnson & de Morais 2006). The A–a gradient is discussed below.

A–a gradient

An A-a gradient (alveolar-arterial) will measure the oxygen transfer across the alveolar membrane into the pulmonary capillaries from the alveoli and the reverse. Most pulmonary diseases will alter the ventilation:perfusion (V/Q) ratio of the lungs. This will lower the amount of oxygen going into the blood, which will then cause the PaO_2 to decrease. A V/Q mismatch can cause the A–a gradient to be elevated.

A–a gradient formula: $[FIO_2 \times (P^B\text{-}47)] - (1.2 \times PaCO_2) - PaO_2$

FIO_2 = fraction of inspired oxygen

P^B = atmospheric pressure (760 mmHg at sea level)

47 is the water vapor pressure in mmHg

1.2 is the respiratory quotient

A simplified A–a gradient formula: $150 - (1.2 \times PaCO_2) - PaO_2$

Normal values for A–a gradient are 5–7 mmHg on a patient breathing 21% oxygen or up to 100 mmHg on a patient breathing 100% oxygen (Haskins 2004). Normal results will exclude pulmonary disease as the reason for the hypoxemia and suggest the reason for hypoxemia is due to hypoventilation or decreased inspired oxygen. If the value is above normal, a V/Q mismatch from pulmonary parenchymal disease or cardiovascular pathology should be suspected (Balakrishnan & King 2014).

PaO_2:FiO_2

PaO_2:FiO_2 is the calculation of choice if the patient is being supplemented with oxygen. A normal level of oxygenation should be calculated at five times the fraction of inspired oxygen (FiO_2). For example, if the patient is breathing 100% oxygen, the PaO_2 should be 500 mmHg.

In the past it had been recommended to classify acute lung injury (ALI) versus ARDS based on the calculated number of this equation. The current recommendation is to classify the degree of ARDS based on when the result of the calculation are:
- 200–300: Mild ARDS
- 100–200: Moderate ARDS
- <100: Severe ARDS

Common causes for an increased PaO_2:FiO_2 ratio or alveolar hypoxia are a diffusion abnormality, V/Q mismatch, or right to left shunt. (Balakrishnan & King 2014).

Right to left shunt

Right to left shunt occurs when both oxygenated and deoxygenated blood returns to the left side of the heart. A small amount of shunting occurs normally in every patient; it is when the shunt is due to lack of ventilation because of atelectasis or consolidation that it becomes pathologic. A right to left shunt is considered a severe form of V/Q mismatch. The cause of hypoxemia in pulmonary diseases such as pulmonary edema, atelectasis, pneumonia, and congenital cardiac abnormalities is due to a right to left shunt amongst other causes (Johnson & de Morais 2006). A patient experiencing a right to left shunt will not return to normal PaO_2 levels on 100% oxygen.

Patients that have diseases associated with respiratory acid-base disturbances should be properly monitored and diagnosed in a timely manner. Treatment of the underlying condition will improve the patient's prognosis. The availability of blood gas analyzers and monitoring equipment in the practice will help improve patient outcomes. Increased knowledge and technical skills will help the technician become a dependable member of the veterinary team.

References

Balakrishnan, A. & King, L. (2014). Update on pulmonary function testing in small animals. *Veterinary Clinics of North America: Small animal practice*. St Louis, MO: Saunders Elsevier: 1–18.

Boothe, D. (2011). Anti-inflammatory drugs. In D. Boothe (ed.), *Small Animal Clinical Pharmacology and Therapeutics*. Philadelphia: W. B. Saunders: 281–311.

Crowe, D. (2009). Oxygen therapy. In: J. Bonagura & D. Twedt (eds), *Kirk's Current Veterinary Therapy XIV*. St. Louis, MO: Saunders Elsevier: 596–603.

de Morais, H. & DiBartola, S. (2009). Acid-base disorders. In: J. Bonagura & D. Twedt (eds), *Kirk's Current Veterinary Therapy XIV*. St. Louis, MO: Saunders Elsevier: 54–61.

DiBartola, S. (2012). *Introduction to Acid-Base Disorders, Fluid, Electrolytes and Acid-Base Disorders in Small Animal Practice*, 4th ed. In: S. P. DiBartola (ed.), St Louis, MO: Saunders Elsevier: 231–52.

Hackett, T. (2009). Tachypnea and hypoxemia, In: D. Silverstein & K. Hopper (eds), *Critical Care Medicine*. St Louis, MO: Saunders Elsevier: 37–40.

Hall, J. (2011a). Pulmonary ventilation. In: J. Hall (ed.), *Guyton and Hall Textbook of Medical Physiology*, 12th ed. Philadelphia: Saunders Elsevier: 465–475.

Hall, J. (2011b). Physical principles of gas exchange diffusion oxygen and carbon dioxide through respiratory membrane. In: J. Hall (ed.), *Guyton and Hall Textbook of Medical Physiology*, 12th ed. Philadelphia: Saunders Elsevier: 485–494.

Hall, J. (2011c). Transport of oxygen and carbon dioxide. In: J. Hall (ed.), *Guyton and Hall Textbook of Medical Physiology*, 12th ed. Philadelphia: Saunders Elsevier: 495–504.

Hall, J. (2011d). Regulation of respiration. In: J. Hall (ed.), *Guyton and Hall Textbook of Medical Physiology*, 12th ed. Philadelphia: Saunders Elsevier: 505–512.

Haskins, S. (2004). Interpretation of blood gas measurements. In: L. King (ed.), *Textbook of Respiratory Disease in Dogs and Cats*. St Louis, MO: Saunders Elsevier: 181–95.

Haskins, S. (2006). Pulmonary physiology: Gas exchange in the awake and anesthetized multidisciplinary review AVECC. *Proceedings from the International Emergency and Critical Care Symposium*, Texas.

Haskins, S. (2007). Mechanical ventilation. *Proceedings of the Latin America Veterinary Emergency and Critical Care Society*, Ecuador.

Heath, D. & Atkins, L. (2012). Respiratory emergencies. In C. Norkus (ed.), *Veterinary Technician Manual for Small Animal Emergency and Critical Care*. Ames, IA: Wiley-Blackwell: 127–50.

Johnson, R. & de Morais, H. A. (2006). Respiratory acid base disorders. In S. P. DiBartola (ed.), *Fluid, Electrolyte and Acid Base Disorders in Small Animal Practice*, 3rd ed. St Louis, MO: Saunders Elsevier: 283–95.

Johnson, R. & de Morais, H. A. (2012). Respiratory acid base disorders. In: S. P. DiBartola (ed.), *Fluid, Electrolyte, and Acid-Base Disorders in Small Animal Practice*, 4th ed. St Louis, MO: W. B. Saunders: 287–301.

McDonnel, W. & Kerr, C. (2007). Respiratory system. In: W. Tranquilli, J. Thurmon, & K. Grimm (eds), *Lumb and Jones Veterinary Anesthesia and Analgesia*, 4th ed. Ames, IA: Blackwell Publishing: 117–154.

Monning, A. (2013). Practical acid base in veterinary patients. *Veterinary Clinics of North America, Small Animal Practice* **43**(6): 1273–86.

Randels, A. (2013). Acid base for beginners. *Proceedings of the International Emergency and Critical Care Symposium*, California.

Tseng, L. & Drobatz, K. (2004). Oxygen supplementation and humidification. In: L. King (ed.), *Textbook of Respiratory Diseases in Dogs and Cats*. St Louis, MO: Saunders Elsevier: 205–213.

CHAPTER 11

Mixed Acid-Base Disorders

Brandee Bean, CVT, VTS (ECC)

Evaluating blood gas results for mixed acid-base disorders can be a daunting task due to the complex nature of these conditions and the confusing and conflicting results reported on a blood gas measurement. A systematic approach makes the results easier to interpret. As discussed in earlier chapters blood gas disorders can be characterized as simple or mixed: simple having one primary disorder and a compensatory response and mixed meaning two or more contributing causes that are not attributed to compensation of the body system alone. As these disorders reflect outward manifestations of multiple disease processes, a thorough patient history and physical exam are necessary to begin evaluation. It is important to learn duration of symptoms, establish pertinent underlying diseases processes, and be aware of any changes in these disease states.

Review and overview of mixed disorders (Figure 11.1)

Acid-base balance represents a fine line between acid production and loss and base production and loss. The body requires the pH to remain within a very narrow range and adjusts for this by retaining or excreting acids or bases in the kidney and retaining or excreting CO_2 in the lungs. The respiratory component is measured with partial pressure of carbon dioxide (pCO_2) and the metabolic with bicarbonate (HCO_3^-) or base excess (BE). PH responds directly with HCO_3^- and inversely with pCO_2. When the body is responding appropriately the lungs will quickly begin to compensate for metabolic changes in pH and the kidneys will more slowly begin to compensate for respiratory changes in pH, and it takes longer for full renal compensation to occur.

A mixed acid-base disorder is present when there is more than one primary acid-base disturbance occurring at the same time in the same patient. These

Acid-Base and Electrolyte Handbook for Veterinary Technicians, First Edition.
Edited by Angela Randels-Thorp and David Liss.
© 2017 John Wiley & Sons, Inc. Published 2017 by John Wiley & Sons, Inc.
Companion website: www.wiley.com/go/liss/electrolytes

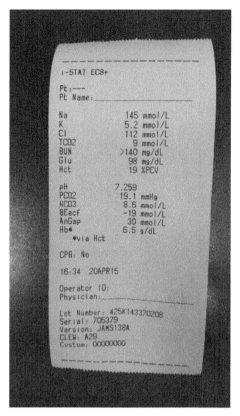

Figure 11.1 Mixed acid-base disorder with a high anion gap acidosis and inappropriate compensation as shown on a cage side chemistry analyzer.

mixed disorders are common in emergent and critical care patients. Mixed disturbances can cause unexpected changes in pH. For instance, if there are two alkalotic processes occurring then the pH can be much higher than a single disorder might produce. It is also imperative to look to the pCO_2 and the HCO_3^- for additional clues to which processes are contributing. If the HCO_3^- is increased and the pCO_2 is decreased then there is a metabolic alkalosis and a respiratory alkalosis present and a mixed disorder is evident.

Compensation (Table 11.1)

So far we have only discussed simple disorders, or ones with a primary acidosis or alkalosis and its corresponding compensation. For any increase or decrease in pCO_2 there should be a compensatory response in HCO_3^-. Respiratory compensation to metabolic disorders begins quickly and metabolic compensation needs much longer to respond to respiratory acid-base disorders. If there is little to no metabolic compensation, it suggests that the respiratory disorder is acute in

Table 11.1 Expected compensatory response to acid-base disorders (Source: Adapted from de Morais & DiBartola 1991)

Disorders	Primary Change	Appropriate Compensation
Metabolic acidosis	Each 1 mEq/L decrease in HCO_3^-	pCO_2 decreases by 0.7 mmHg
Metabolic alkalosis	Each 1 mEq/L increase in HCO_3^-	pCO_2 increases by 0.7 mmHg
Acute respiratory acidosis	Each 1 mmHg increase in pCO_2	HCO_3 increases by 0.15 mEq/L
Chronic respiratory acidosis	Each 1 mmHg increase in pCO_2	HCO_3 increases by 0.35 mEq/L
Long-standing respiratory acidosis	Each 1 mmHg increase in pCO_2	HCO_3 increases by 0.55 mEq/L
Acute respiratory alkalosis	Each 1 mmHg decrease in pCO_2	HCO_3 decreases by 0.25 mEq/L
Chronic respiratory alkalosis	Each 1 mmHg decrease in pCO_2	HCO_3 decreases by 0.55 mEq/L

nature. However, if compensation seems complete then it is likely that the disease is of a more chronic nature. Chronic respiratory disorders in dogs are those lasting longer than 2–5 days. Long-standing respiratory diseases are those lasting longer than 30 days (de Morais & DiBartola 1991). In order to assess if there is a mixed disorder one must evaluate for expected compensation, and consider the patient status and disease process. Calculating the expected compensatory response begins to elucidate whether one is dealing with a single or a mixed disorder. We will first deal with respiratory disorders.

Compensatory responses of respiratory disorders

Respiratory alkalosis

Respiratory alkalosis can be divided into two forms: acute and chronic disease with differing expected metabolic responses. In acute respiratory alkalosis for every 1 mmHg decrease in pCO_2 there should be an HCO_3^- decrease of 0.25 mEq/L. In chronic respiratory alkalosis for every 1 mmHg decrease in pCO_2 there should be a decrease of 0.55 mEq/L in HCO_3^-. The equation for this is:

$$\text{Expected } HCO_3^- = \left(\text{midpoint } HCO_3^-\right) - [(\text{midpoint } pCO_2 - \text{patient } pCO_2) \times \text{compensation rate}]$$

Refer to examples in Table 11.2 for midpoint values. Given an acute respiratory alkalosis, pH 7.5, HCO_3^- 19 mEq/L, and pCO_2 30 mmHg:

$$\begin{aligned} \text{Expected } HCO_3^- &= 22.5 \text{ mEq / L} - (37.5 \text{ mmHg} - 30 \text{ mmHg}) \times 0.25 \text{ mEq / L} \\ &= 22.5 \text{ mEq / L} - 7.5 \times 0.25 \text{ mEq / L} \\ &= 22.5 \text{ mEq / L} - 1.875 \text{ mEq / L} \end{aligned}$$

Expected $HCO_3^- = 20.625$ mEq/L +/− 2. This shows appropriate compensation.

Table 11.2 Example cases

	Case 1	Case 2	Case 3	Normal range	Midpoint
pH	7.397	7.31	7.19	7.35–7.45	7.4
pCO_2	47.1 mmHg	33 mmHg	47.8 mmHg	34–40 mmHg	37.5 mmHg
HCO_3^-	28.9 mmol/L	18.7 mmol/L	19.2 mmol/L	20–24 mmol/L	22.5 mmol/L
BE	4	−6	−7	(−5)–(0)	
Na	160 mmol/L	141 mmol/L	139 mmol/L	139–150 mmol/L	
Cl	121 mmol/L	111 mmol/L	95 mmol/L	106–127 mmol/L	
K	4.5 mmol/L	3.9 mmol/L	5.1 mmol/L	3.4–4.9 mmol/L	

Respiratory acidosis

For respiratory acidosis expected compensation can be further divided into acute, chronic, and long-standing disorders. In acute respiratory acidosis, for every 1 mmHg increase in pCO_2 there should be an increase in HCO_3^- of 0.15 mEq/L. In chronic respiratory acidosis, each 1 mmHg increase in pCO_2 should result in a 0.35 mEq/L increase in HCO_3^-. In long-standing respiratory acidosis, for every 1 mmHg increase in pCO_2 there should be a corresponding 0.55 mEq/L increase in HCO_3^-. The equation for this is:

$$\text{Expected } HCO_3^- = \left(\text{midpoint } HCO_3^-\right) + \left[\left(\text{patient } pCO_2 - \text{midpoint } pCO_2\right) \times \text{compensation rate}\right]$$

Refer to examples in Table 11.2 for midpoint values. Given an acute respiratory acidosis, pH 7.32, HCO_3^- 26 mEq/L, and pCO_2 55 mmHg:

$$\begin{aligned}
\text{Expected } HCO_3^- &= 22.5\,\text{mEq}/\text{L} + \left(55\,\text{mmHg} - 37.5\,\text{mmHg}\right) \times 0.15\,\text{mEq}/\text{L} \\
&= 22.5\,\text{mEq}/\text{L} + 17.5 \times 0.15\,\text{mEq}/\text{L} \\
&= 22.5\,\text{mEq}/\text{L} + 2.625\,\text{mEq}/\text{L}
\end{aligned}$$

Expected $HCO_3^- = 25.125$ mEq/L +/− 2. This shows appropriate compensation.

For respiratory disorders you should allow an error margin of +/−2 mEq/L. As you can see the more established the respiratory disease the more complete the compensation and in the case of chronic and possibly long-standing respiratory disorders it may even be possible for compensation to return the pH to normal which is not the case in acute respiratory disorders or in metabolic disorders of any kind (de Morais & DiBartola 1991).

Compensatory responses of metabolic disorders

Metabolic acidosis

In metabolic acidosis of dogs for each 1 mEq/L decrease in HCO_3^- there should be a pCO_2 decrease of 0.7 mmHg, but in experiments with cats there does not seem to be any pCO_2 compensation. The equation for this is:

$$\text{Expected } pCO_2 = \text{midpoint } pCO_2 - \left[\left(\text{midpoint } HCO_3^-\right) - \left(\text{patient } HCO_3^-\right)\right] \times$$
$$\text{compensation rate}$$

Refer to examples in Table 11.2 for midpoint values. Given a metabolic acidosis, pH 7.3, HCO_3^- 18.5 mEq/L, and pCO_2 33 mmHg.

$$\text{Expected } pCO_2 = 37.5\,\text{mmHg} - \left(22.5\,\text{mEq}/\text{L} - 18.5\,\text{mEq}/\text{L}\right) \times 0.7\,\text{mmHg}$$
$$= 37.5\,\text{mmHg} - 4 \times 0.7\,\text{mmHg}$$
$$= 37.5\,\text{mmHg} - 2.8\,\text{mmHg}$$

Expected $pCO_2 = 34.7$ mmHg +/− 3. This shows appropriate compensation.

Metabolic alkalosis

With metabolic alkalosis for each 1 mEq/L increase in HCO_3^- there should be a pCO_2 increase of 0.7 mmHg. The equation for this is:

$$\text{Expected } pCO_2 = \text{midpoint } pCO_2 + \left[\left(\text{patient } HCO_3^-\right) - \left(\text{midpoint } HCO_3^-\right)\right] \times$$
$$\text{compensation rate}$$

Refer to examples in Table 11.2 for midpoint values. Given a metabolic alkalosis, pH 7.49, HCO_3^- 26 mEq/L, and pCO_2 41 mmHg.

$$\text{Expected } pCO_2 = 37.5\,\text{mmHg} + \left(26\,\text{mEq}/\text{L} - 22.5\,\text{mEq}/\text{L}\right) \times 0.7\,\text{mmHg}$$
$$= 37.5\,\text{mmHg} + 3.5 \times 0.7\,\text{mmHg}$$
$$= 37.5\,\text{mmHg} + 2.45\,\text{mmHg}$$

Expected $pCO_2 = 39.95$ mmHg +/− 3. This shows appropriate compensation. When calculating compensation for metabolic disorders an error margin of +/− 3 mmHg should be expected. Most of the compensation calculations may or may not be accurate in cats as a very limited number of studies have been published and none was performed in awake, adult, sick cats. So compensation formulas should be used with caution in cats. Even in dogs these are only guidelines to help the investigation (de Morais & DiBartola 1991). After evaluation for possible compensation is complete, if the investigation yields an inappropriate compensatory response this is most likely a mixed disorder.

> **Box 11.1** Clues to help identify mixed acid-base disorders
>
> - Normal pH in the presence of abnormal pCO_2 or HCO_3^-
> - Inappropriate compensation despite appropriate time lapse
> - Acidemia in a known alkalemic disease process
> - Alkalemia in a known acidemic disease process
> - HCO_3^- and pCO_2 changing in opposite directions
> - Anion gap without corresponding change in HCO_3^-
> - Hyperchloremia not following corresponding changes in HCO_3^-

The anion gap and chloride's role (Box 11.1)

Anion gap
Other tools exist to assist the veterinary technician in evaluating for mixed acid-base disorders. The anion gap is one such tool. Many analyzers calculate the anion gap for the user, but it can also be calculated by hand. The anion gap doesn't actually exist physiologically, because in reality there is no gap of anions. It is just that cations are more readily seen in current laboratory measures as opposed to the anions that exist but are not usually measured on standard blood work in most hospitals. The anion gap equation is the major cations minus the usually tested anions. Generally the anion gap should be less than 20. If there is a high anion gap then a primary metabolic acidosis is present in addition to whatever other processes are seen. The equation used to obtain the anion gap measurement follows:

$$AG = \left(\left[Na^+ \right] + \left[K^+ \right] \right) - \left(\left[HCO_3^- \right] + \left[Cl^- \right] \right)$$

$\left[Na^+ \right]$ = sodium, $\left[K^+ \right]$ = potassium, $\left[HCO_3^- \right]$ = bicarbonate, and $\left[Cl^- \right]$ = Chloride

Contributing factors in anion gap acidosis in clinical practice often follow the MUDPILES acronym and can be exogenous, such as ethanol (from alcohol ingestion and also from the fermentation of sugars and yeast), ethylene and propylene glycol ingestions (in conventional and in "safer" antifreeze products respectively), and salicylate (aspirin), as well as endogenous causes such as ketones, lactic acid, and uremic acids. Ketones can be evaluated using color changing strips that can test either the urine or the serum. Handheld lactate monitors are now available and affordable.

Using the anion gap to evaluate for mixed disorders
The change in anion gap should be approximately the same as the change of the HCO_3^- if a simple disorder is present. If a mixed disorder is present the changes may deviate from what is expected. Anion gap measurements become less useful

in the face of hypoalbuminemia because it hides the presence of anions. A high anion gap is associated with a primary metabolic acidosis no matter what the pH or pCO_2 results are.

Effect of chloride

Chloride changes occur as a result of alterations in pH or water balance. Typically with water balance abnormalities sodium and chloride shift in parallel and often in the same quantity because chloride actively and passively follows sodium in order to maintain osmolality, whereas with acid-base abnormalities a disparity between the two might exist. Hyperchloremia without a corresponding hyper-natremia often occurs in metabolic acidosis because of the strong ion difference, and inversely hypochloremia without a parallel hyponatremia occurs with metabolic alkalosis. Hyperchloremia should accompany a corresponding decrease in HCO_3^- because of the chloride shift that occurs when chloride enters the cell and HCO_3^- moves out of the cell. (More can be read about strong ion difference in Chapter 12.) Mixed disorders are highly possible if this change does not occur.

Various clinicopathologic findings can indicate underlying acid-base disorders. Hypernatremia, hypokalemia, and hypoalbuminemia may be associated with metabolic alkalosis. Conversely, hyponatremia, hyperalbuminemia, hyperkalemia, and hyperphosphatemia can be related to metabolic acidosis. Evaluating sodium, potassium, chloride, and bicarbonate levels is of the utmost importance when searching for the etiology of a mixed acid-base disorder.

Steps in evaluating for mixed acid-base disorders

1 Assess the pH. When evaluating mixed acid-base disorders it is crucial to start with assessing the pH to determine whether you are dealing with an acidosis or an alkalosis. It is imperative to note that even if the pH is normal that does not exclude the possibility of a mixed disorder and it is still necessary to evaluate the pCO_2 and HCO_3^-. For instance, a mixed disorder with metabolic acidosis and respiratory alkalosis combined could result in a normal pH.

2 Determine the origin of the disorder. Evaluate whether the disorder is metabolic or respiratory in origin. If pCO_2, HCO_3^-, or BE are abnormal but the pH is normal then there is a mixed disorder present. This would occur if an acidosis and an alkalosis were working against each other to produce a normal pH. The only exception to this is that chronic and possibly long-standing respiratory diseases can sometimes cause enough compensation to return a patient's pH to normal.

3 Evaluate appropriate compensation. The most critical factor in evaluating secondary compensation to a primary disorder is the length of time that the disorder has been present. Adequate time needs to have elapsed for compensation to occur. When compensation is responsible for a change in pH, the

pCO_2 and HCO_3^- should always increase together or decrease together. For example, in a metabolic acidosis with respiratory compensation the primary change is a decrease in HCO_3^- and the compensatory change is a lesser decrease in pCO_2. If, however, the HCO_3^- decreases and the pCO_2 increases then this cannot be a compensatory response to a simple disorder. It must instead be two separate disorders at work. In this example it would be a metabolic acidosis and a respiratory acidosis causing a mixed disorder and most likely the additive effects would make the pH dangerously low. It is also important to remember that although the clinical picture might show results consistent with a simple disorder and appropriate compensation, a mixed disorder could still be present.

4 Identify other contributing factors. As shown above, many other factors can affect acid-base in dogs and cats. Electrolytes (especially chloride), measured and unmeasured anions, and albumin (which is a weak acid) can all alter pH and need to be taken into account when deciding whether a mixed disorder is present. Also be aware when dealing with a known disorder, such as diabetic ketoacidosis, if the pH change is opposite from what would be expected then further evaluations should be made for a mixed disorder. Other factors may need to be taken into account, such as patient history, other laboratory results, and physical exam findings.

Effects of mixed disorders on pH

Mixed acid-base disorders in combination can have different effects on the pH. In general, two acid-base conditions of the same category (acidosis or alkalosis) will have an additive effect on the abnormal pH and will both contribute to an increasingly acidotic or alkalotic pH. That is to say that if there are two acidotic processes then they will enhance each other, sometimes creating dangerously low pH. When an acidotic process and alkalotic process are combined the pH will depend on the severity of each disorder. PH can be high, low, or normal, but in general they will neutralize each other to at least some extent. In these cases the pH derangement from normal is usually less severe. In triple mixed disorders the pH could lie anywhere on the spectrum depending on the severity of the different processes.

Specific diseases known to cause mixed disorders (Box 11.2)

Some disease processes tend to cause mixed acid-base disorders. Therefore it is valuable to closely assess laboratory values in these cases. Continued monitoring of acid-base values in these disease processes can be lifesaving because in the

---

> **Box 11.2** Diseases commonly presenting with mixed acid-base disorders
>
> - Diabetic ketoacidosis
> - Gastric dilatation volvulus
> - Renal failure
> - Cardiopulmonary arrest
> - Congestive heart failure
> - Heatstroke
> - Sepsis
> - Parvo virus

course of treating one abnormality it is possible to cause more physiologic harm as the other disorder continues untreated.

Gastric dilatation volvulus (GDV) is one disease that can present with many different mixed acid-base disorders. By the very nature of its complex physiology it is not unusual for GDV patients to have two or more mixed acid-base disorders. This condition can cause metabolic acidosis from hyperlactatemia and respiratory acidosis from impaired ventilation. These two acid-base abnormalities have the additive effect described above and can make the pH plummet. These patients can also present with metabolic alkalosis from loss of gastric acid. Metabolic alkalosis and metabolic acidosis are also possible from loss of gastric acid and increased lactate levels. Depending on the duration of symptoms, the pH can be nearly normal due to the competing effects of an alkalosis and acidosis. Patients with GDV can even have triple disorders caused by any of the above. In these cases the HCO_3^- and pH can be high, low, or normal and pCO_2 will be increased beyond normal compensation. Rapid interpretation of blood gas abnormalities and identification of underlying causes will exert a positive effect on the patient's outcome.

Parvovirus is another disease that can present with multiple mixed acid-base disorders. With vomiting, diarrhea, hypoalbuminemia, and sepsis it becomes easy to see that these patients may present with respiratory alkalosis, from pain and inflammation, and metabolic acidosis from diarrhea, shock, or hypovolemia. A triple disorder is also possible when metabolic alkalosis from vomiting is added. Frequent monitoring for pain, electrolytes, and blood gas values are very important in the proper management of these patients.

Multiple disease processes in some patients can increase the likelihood of mixed acid-base disorders where the individual diseases have an underlying acid-base condition that contributes equally to a mixed disorder. For instance, it is not unusual for a feline patient with diabetes ketoacidosis (DKA) to also have concurrent renal failure. To further complicate matters, many are anemic. Diabetic ketoacidosis or renal failure alone can cause a high anion gap acidosis from ketonemia or uremia and if there is vomiting from either the renal failure or DKA it can become complicated with a metabolic alkalosis from hypochloremia.

Anemia and stress can both cause hyperventilation and respiratory alkalosis. The patient could easily have a mixed or triple acid-base disorder. So it is easy to see how the mixed acid-base disorders could multiply.

Treatment

Treatment of mixed acid-base disorders involves rapid evaluation of the disorder and identifying which etiology is the most urgent. With multiple disorders at play the veterinary technician and veterinarian must be aware of all possible causes as neglecting one cause to treat another could make the situation worse. In some patients, the combination of initial treatments and compensatory mechanisms are enough to correct the acid-base imbalance. Treatment of disorders with very high or low pH will need to be treated more aggressively than those that are closer to normal (DiBartola 2006). It is also imperative to monitor for iatrogenic acidosis and alkalosis during treatment. Remember that some of our fluid therapies are rich in chloride and sodium and most are acidifying to differing degrees.

Severe life-threatening acidosis can be treated with intravenous fluids and potentially sodium bicarbonate. Sodium bicarbonate therapy has mostly fallen out of favor but when it is used in mixed acid-base disorders blood gases and electrolytes should be monitored carefully during infusion. When sodium bicarbonate is used to treat an acidemia, it is converted into carbonic acid which disassociate into water and CO_2. If there is a respiratory acidosis present and the patient is unable to eliminate the CO_2 it can dangerously worsen the acidemia (Adams & Polzin 1989). Sodium bicarbonate also shifts the oxygen dissociation curve causing decreased oxygenation to tissues including the brain (Plumb 2011). The resultant effect of sodium bicarbonate therapy can be especially hard to predict in mixed disorders, where overcorrecting the pH can create another possibly worse problem. In addition, treatment of the primary disease process (DKA, for example) might negatively impact the acid-base disorders. If a patient already has a mixed respiratory and metabolic acidosis and is given pharmacologic agents that depress the central nervous system, hypoventilation may result, worsening the acidosis. Ventilator support may be necessary if this is the case.

Sampling errors

Correct blood sampling techniques are critical to ensure accurate results. In most patients only small differences are seen between arterial and venous samples. Arterial samples are the gold standard for blood gases, but for acid-base analysis venous samples are usually adequate as long as normal venous values are used for your reference ranges. The exception is when there is poor peripheral perfusion such as during shock states and cardiopulmonary resuscitation. Arterial samples are less affected by blood stasis. Poor perfusion can falsely elevate pCO_2 and lactic acid and decrease pH. Central samples are therefore more accurate for assessment. Care should be taken that the patient experience as little stress as possible during restraint and blood drawing because thrashing, pain, and fear can all cause hyperventilation and derangements in pCO_2 and pH. Anemia and hypovolemia can also affect values. Samples with greater than 10% heparin can falsely decreases HCO_3^- and pCO_2. Samples should be free from air bubbles. Blood should be analyzed as soon as possible (no more than within 15–30 minutes) because the pCO_2 increases and pH decreases in a resting sample. Core body temperature also affects sample results. Hypothermic patients will have falsely decreased pH and increased pCO_2. Conversely, hyperthermic patients will have falsely increased pH and increased pCO_2. The changes are, in general, relatively small for mild increases or decreases in temperature but for severe changes in core body temperature the errors can add up. Most analyzers allow you to input body temperature to correct for the discrepancy, although the actual clinical significance is debatable.

Conclusion

Acid-base analysis for mixed disorders is complicated but can be simplified with a systematic approach that encompasses physical exam, patient history, and laboratory results. Treatment hinges on finding the underlying disease processes and addressing them. Errors in calculation and sampling should be assessed as well. The best way to become better at assessment of mixed disorders is to evaluate as many as possible and discuss possible causes and treatments with the rest of your veterinary team.

References

Adams, L. & Polzin, D. J. (1989). Mixed acid-base disorders. *Veterinary Clinics of North America: Small Animal Practice* **19**(2): 307–26.
de Morais, H. A. & DiBartola, S. (1991). Ventilatory and metabolic compensation in dogs with acid-base disturbances. *Journal of Veterinary Emergency and Critical Care* **1**(2): 39–49.
DiBartola, S. (2006). *Fluid, Electrolyte, and Acid-Base Disorders in Small Animal Practice*, 3rd ed. St Louis, MO: Elsevier.
Plumb, D. C. (2011). *Plumb's Veterinary Drug Handbook*, 7th ed. St Louis, MO: PharmaVet Inc.

CHAPTER 12

Strong Ion Approach to Acid-Base

Angela Randels-Thorp, CVT, VTS (ECC, SAIM)

The importance of acid-base assessment in the critical care setting cannot be overstated. Clinical assessment of acid-base has been advocated for critically ill veterinary patients for some time. However, thoughts surrounding the approach to the acid-base status of a patient have shifted. The original or traditional approach involved utilizing Henderson–Hasselbalch methodology and has been the standard used in clinical practice for years (Chawla 2008). In 1983, Peter Stewart introduced an alternate concept to assess clinical acid-base disturbances by employing the strong ion difference. The strong ion model more clearly explains the relationship between electrolytes and changes seen in acid-base status, whereas the traditional approach tends to lead one to the conclusion that electrolyte changes occur secondary to the changes in acid-base status rather than being directly related to them. This is only one difference in the two approaches. Henderson–Hasselbalch and strong ion theory are equally useful when plasma protein (albumin), phosphate, and globulin concentrations are normal (Constable 1999). Both approaches have advantages and limitations in their use. Is one approach better? What is more useful in clinical practice? Is the strong ion approach practical for using in a clinical setting?

Henderson–Hasselbalch: Overview of traditional approach to acid-base

The traditional approach utilizes pH, pCO_2, and HCO_3^- to evaluate acid-base status in patients (Kovacic 2009). If hydrogen ions are increased, there is an acidosis. If hydrogen ions are decreased, there is an alkalosis. Changes in pCO_2 are

Acid-Base and Electrolyte Handbook for Veterinary Technicians, First Edition.
Edited by Angela Randels-Thorp and David Liss.
© 2017 John Wiley & Sons, Inc. Published 2017 by John Wiley & Sons, Inc.
Companion website: www.wiley.com/go/liss/electrolytes

considered similar in both approaches so are considered briefly in this chapter. The traditional theory makes it easy to conclude that hydrogen [H⁺] and bicarbonate [HCO₃⁻] ions are the root of all metabolic acid-base issues. Yet in alkaline states, there are little to no hydrogen ions present and alkalosis presents a clinical problem for the patient. How so? Additionally, it is known that changing the temperature of water changes the number of hydrogen ions, yet water always remains acid-base neutral. Henderson–Hasselbalch's approach to acid-base cannot explain this phenomenon. This theory suggests that hydrogen ion concentrations are an independent variable as opposed to a dependent one. Additionally, this approach does not explain that the underlying factors indicate the changes are represented as a pH number and are dependent on concentrations of other ions and independent factors. The whys of the issue are not fully explained. Instead only the symptoms, or the result, of the underlying changes occurring are looked at. The Stewart approach, on the other hand, takes this into account.

Advantages of the traditional approach are that it is easy to calculate and utilize in clinical practice. Because it has been widely used, it has become well understood. In patients with normal protein and phosphate concentrations, this approach is adequate to assess an approximation of what is occurring systemically. However, the approach has several drawbacks: it does not take into account changes in protein and phosphorus, anion gap calculations lack specificity and sensitivity, effects of temperature on pH are not explained, dependence of pK_1 on pH is not explained, it demonstrates log pCO_2 and pH to have a linear relationship, it leads one to conclude that changes in electrolytes are secondary, and it does not take into account changes in protein or phosphate concentrations and the effect on pH.

Stewart's strong ion approach to acid-base

In order to fully understand the strong ion approach to acid-base we must re-evaluate the definitions of neutral, alkaline, acid, acidic, and base. The following definitions support the theory of strong ion:

Acid-base neutral = hydrogen ion concentration is equal to its hydroxyl ion

$$concentration; \left[H^+\right] = \left[OH^-\right]$$

Acidic = hydrogen ion concentration is greater than its hydroxyl ion

$$concentration; \left[H^+\right] > \left[OH^-\right]$$

Alkaline = hydrogen ion concentration is less than its hydroxyl ion
concentration; $\left[H^+ \right] < \left[OH^- \right]$

Acid = a substance is an acid if it brings about an increase in hydrogen ion
concentration

Base = a substance is a base if it brings about a decrease in hydrogen ion
concentration

These definitions vary from Bronsted and Lowry's definition of an acid being
a proton-donor and a base being a proton-acceptor (DiBartola 2006). Stewart
asserts that the above definitions are more useful for considering acid-base
balance in living beings (Kellum & Elbers 2009).

Stewart's approach takes into account dependent variables such as hydrogen
ions [H+], hydroxide ions [OH-], bicarbonate [HCO_3^-], carbon trioxide [CO_3^{2-}],
other weak acids [HA], and weak ions [A-] (Grogono 2011). A vital concept of
Stewart's approach is independent variables such as carbon dioxide [pCO_2], total
weak non-volatile acids [A_{TOT}], and net strong ion difference [SID] (Worthley
1999). Consideration of these independent variables is necessary to utilize the
strong ion approach as Stewart hypothesized in a series of simultaneous equations to determine their influence, being:

1 $[H^+] \times [OH^-] = K_w$ (water dissociation equilibrium)
2 $[H^+] \times [A^-] = K_A \times [HA]$ (weak acid)
3 $[HA] + [A^-] = [A_{TOT}]$ (conservation of mass for "A")
4 $[H^+] \times [HCO_3^-] = K_c \times pCO_2$ (bicarbonate ion formation equilibrium)
5 $[H^+] \times [CO_3^{2-}] = K_3 \times [HCO_3^-]$ (carbonate ion formation equilibrium)
6 $[SID] + [H^+] - [HCO_3^-] - [A^-] - [CO_3^{2-}] - [OH^-] = 0$ (electrical neutrality) (Nickson
2012)

Because Stewart's approach relies heavily on mechanical approaches and calculations, it has been one of the major disadvantages of using it in clinical practice.
Additional calculations utilized in this approach include:

[SID]: The difference between the sums of concentrations of the strong cations
and strong ions:

$$[SID] = \left(\left[Na^+ \right] + \left[K^+ \right] + \left[Ca^{2+} \right] + \left[MG^{2+} \right] \right) - \left(\left[Cl^- \right] - \left[\text{other strong anions} \right] \right)$$

[A_{TOT}]: The total plasma concentration of the weak non-volatile acids, inorganic
phosphate, serum proteins, and albumin: $[A_{TOT}] = [P_{iTOT}] + [Pr_{TOT}] + \text{albumin}$.

[pCO_2]: Mechanisms of effects of pCO_2 on acid-base status are considered
below. To further understand these concepts, we must look closer at
the independent variables and their effects, namely [SID] and [A_{tot}]
(Figure 12.1).

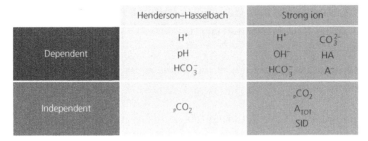

Figure 12.1 Variables in A-B evaluation.

Strong ion difference [SID]

The SID is the sum of all strong base cation concentrations minus the sum of all the strong acid anion concentrations. In veterinary patients, the [SID] is almost always positive and approximately +40 mEq/L (normal ranges of SID are 54.5– 33.5 mEq/L theoretically), which accounts for the slight alkalinity in normal patients (pH ~ 7.35–7.45). Whenever [SID] is positive, as described in the definitions above, we can conclude that the following is true: $[OH^-] > [H^+]$. Strong ions do not have a direct effect on pH but rather act as a positive unit of charge. Therefore, when [SID] is positive, $[H^+]$ is very small (the effects of $[A_{TOT}]$ on $[H^+]$ and pH will be considered in the next section). In this way changes in SID affect the patient's acid-base status (Table 12.1).

Strong ions completely dissociate in a solution and comprise buffer and non-buffer ions. SID is the difference between strong cations and strong ions (anions). Any substance that dissociates in water to form ions, either weak or strong, is an electrolyte. The strong ions considered in calculating SID are sodium (Na^+), potassium (K^+), calcium (Ca_2^+), magnesium (Mg_2^+), chloride (Cl^-), lactate, ß-hydroxybutyrate, acetoacetate, and sulfate (SO_4^{2-}). [Abbreviated $SID = (Na+K)-(Cl)$] (Table 12.2). Changes in concentrations of Na^+, Cl^-, and SO_4^{2-} have the most effect on altering acid-base balance by increasing or decreasing SID. An increase in SID, by increased sodium or decreased chloride, will result in a strong ion metabolic alkalosis. A decrease in SID, by decreased sodium or increasing chloride, will result in a strong ion metabolic acidosis. There are two main reasons a change in SID will occur.

1 There will be a change in free water content causing a change in concentration; or

2 Change in strong ions (sodium or chloride primarily).

The kidneys play a large role in maintaining the [SID] by either filtering or reabsorbing Cl^-, Na^+, or K^+. Every Cl^- filtered causes an increase in [SID], causing a shift in pH moving toward alkalosis. Every Na^+ or K^+ not reabsorbed will decrease the [SID], resulting in a shift toward acidosis. Aldosterone also plays a large role in maintaining balance of these electrolytes. The kidneys will compensate for changes in [SID] effectively shifting $[H^+]$ back toward normal.

Table 12.1 SID and effect on acid-base status

SID	Acid-Base Status
Increased (>0)	Alkalosis
Decreased (<0)	Acidosis
Normal	~40 mEq/L

Table 12.2 List of major cations and anions

Cations	Anions
Na^+	Cl^-
K^+	Other strong anions
Ca_2^+	
Mg_2^+	

The gastrointestinal (GI) tract is also an important regulator of strong ion balance. The gastric mucosa removes Cl^- from the plasma into the GI lumen, resulting in gastric acid. This action increases the [SID] in the plasma. [H^+] decreases correspondingly. The pancreas, duodenum, jejunum, ileum, and colon all play a role in maintaining the [SID] rate of absorption of Cl^-, Na^+, and K^+.

SID and alkalosis

An increase in sodium or decrease in chloride can lead to metabolic alkalosis. This occurs due to two mechanisms:

1 Changes in free water in the plasma, or concentration alkalosis; or
2 Hypochloremic alkalosis (relative to plasma-sodium content).

When water decreases, or there is a deficit, a concentration alkalosis may occur. In these cases, hypernatremia or hyperalbuminemia are noted clinically. This occurs in cases of free water or hypotonic fluid loss such as diabetes insipidus, water deprivation, vomiting, or post-obstructive diuresis. The water loss results in an increase in SID which results in a change in ph, or alkalosis. Concentration alkalosis may also occur due to excessive sodium gain (hypertonic saline administration, hyperadrenocorticism) resulting in hypernatremia.

Hypochloremic alkalosis is termed to be either chloride-responsive or chloride-resistant. Hypochloremic alkalosis that does not improve with chloride administration is termed chloride-resistant. Chloride-responsive hypochloremic alkalosis occurs when either water content is normal and chloride decreases or there is a relative decrease in the chloride:sodium ratio, such as in patients that are given solutions containing more sodium than chloride (e.g. sodium bicarbonate). This may also occur when chloride is lost in excess of sodium (e.g. patients with upper gastric vomiting or diuretic therapies). Neither of these pathologies permits the Cl⁻ to be returned to the plasma, thus resulting in an overall decrease. Chloride-resistant hypochloremic alkalosis may occur in patients with hyper-adrenocorticism or hyperaldosteronism. This is due to increased levels of cortisol or aldosterone which cause sodium retention by activating type I renal miner-alocorticoid receptors in the kidneys. These patients have excessively high levels of these hormones, therefore causing sodium retention. Such retention changes the ratio of sodium to chloride, resulting in hypochloremia, a shift in SID, and subsequent metabolic alkalosis.

Treatment of these forms of alkalosis is aimed at treating the underlying cause and supplementing chloride to correct the SID. Therefore, intravenous fluids containing chloride should be administered in these cases. Anti-emetics should be used if vomiting is a major cause of the hypochloremia. Administration of diuretics, if used, should be discontinued. It is important to note that chloride levels will not correct without potassium supplementation in patients with chloride-responsive metabolic alkalosis. Chloride-resistant forms will not improve with chloride and potassium supplementation alone. These patients must have their underlying disease process addressed and treated in order to resolve their metabolic alkalosis.

SID and acidosis

In terms of SID, acidosis may occur when there is a decrease in SID. Any decrease in SID will result in a metabolic acidosis. Three main mechanisms can cause this change:

1 a decrease in sodium or dilutional acidosis
2 an increase in chloride
3 an increase in other strong anions resulting in an organic acidosis.

Dilutional acidosis will be noted clinically by the presence of hyponatremia. This condition may occur with hypervolemia, such as in cases of severe liver disease or congestive heart failure. Patients with dilutional acidosis may also be normovolemic, experiencing a gain in water from hypotonic fluid administration or psychogenic polydipsia. Patients experiencing a dilutional acidosis with hypovolemia undergo a loss of hypertonic fluids by diarrhea, vomiting, third spacing, or by administration of diuretics. Patients with hypoadrenocorticism may also experience dilutional acidosis with hypovolemia. Therapy for dilutional acidosis involves treating the underlying cause and normalizing sodium osmolality levels.

Hyperchloremic acidosis can occur when the loss of sodium is greater than the loss of chloride, retention of chloride, or administration of fluids containing more chloride than sodium (e.g. KCl, 0.9% NaCl) (Kellum & Elbers 2009). Increased levels of chloride decrease SID and result in acidosis. Patients that have been hospitalized on 0.9% NaCl commonly experience hyperchloremic acidosis. Thus, treatment must be aimed at treating the underlying cause of the disorder. Patients with hyperchloremic acidosis should have plasma pH levels monitored closely. A patient with hyperchloremic acidosis and a pH of <7.2 should be given sodium bicarbonate. While sodium bicarbonate use is controversial in the majority of cases, this is one instance that its use is recommended. According to strong ion theory, pH will improve, not necessarily by the administration of the bicarbonate itself but by increasing plasma sodium levels which, in turn, increases SID. As usual, caution should be taken to monitor the level of consciousness and ventilator status of the patient receiving this type of therapy.

Organic acidosis may result from accumulated-acquired or accumulated-organic anions. Common causes of SID acidosis from increased unmeasured strong anions are attributed to organic acids such as acetoacetate or ß-hydroxybutyrate as in cases of diabetic ketoacidosis (DKA), lactic acidosis (heatstroke or shock), or toxicity (ethylene glycol). Sulfate (SO_4^{2-}) is another example of accumulated organic acidosis that occurs in cases of acute kidney injury or chronic disease.

Affects of [A_{TOT}]

[A_{TOT}] is determined by the total plasma concentrations of inorganic phosphate and serum proteins, most notably albumin, as noted in the calculation above. These collectively serve as weak acids that result in changes to the pH when major concentration changes occur. These weak acids frequently serve as buffers in the Stewart approach. On the other hand, Henderson–Hasselbalch does not consider the effects of plasma proteins and phosphates. This is one of the main differences between traditional and strong ion theory. Stewart considers these weak acids to be important as it has been found that decreases in plasma proteins (hypoproteinemia) result in an increase of base excess and alkalemia, and increased phosphate levels contribute to acidemia. An example of this is a patient with kidney disease. These patients experience metabolic acidosis in part due to high levels of phosphate. Thus, changes in A_{TOT} occur due to changes in plasma free water content, and increases or decreases in albumin, globulin, or phosphate.

Non-volatile buffer ion alkalosis

Non-volatile buffer ion alkalosis occurs due to hypoproteinemia. Normal levels of phosphate exist at such low amounts that no decrease in phosphate is enough to contribute to an alkalosis. In human medicine, hypoalbuminemia results in increased pH due to metabolic alkalosis. However, it seems unclear whether low albumin levels directly result in alkalosis in animal patients. Some patients with hypoalbuminemia experience hyperventilation, which may contribute to the alkalosis. Additionally, it has been noted that patients with hypoalbuminemia experience an increase in concentration of chloride, which can decrease the SID, causing an alkalosis as well. Hypoalbuminemia may occur in patients due to decreased production, extracorporeal losses, or sequestration. Patients with non-volatile ion buffer alkalosis due to hypoalbuminemia and decreased $[A_{TOT}]$ have been noted in the critical care setting with disease processes such as chronic liver disease, malnutrition, response to inflammation, protein-losing nephropathy or enteropathies, and inflammatory effusions or vasculitis.

Non-volatile ion buffer acidosis

Acidosis may occur due to increases in hyperphosphatemia induced $[A_{TOT}]$. It is rare for hyperalbuminemia to progress to acidosis, but, as noted above, high phosphate levels in chronic or acute kidney disease or injury may result in hyperphosphatemia occurring to a degree that it is a large contributor to metabolic acidosis (note: acidosis in kidney disease patients is frequently multifactorial). Hypertonic sodium phosphate enemas have been documented to cause acidosis by increasing plasma phosphate concentrations. Treatment should thus be focused on the underlying cause. If sodium bicarbonate is administered, it aids in resolving the acidosis by shifting phosphorus into cells and out of the extracellular fluid space (plasma).

Carbon dioxide and strong ion approach

CO_2 is a byproduct of the metabolism of fat and carbohydrates in the body and is considered a volatile acid (volatile = readily vaporized). On the other hand, gaseous CO_2 is soluble in water. CO_2 is considered an acid because it combines with H_2O in the presence of carbonic anhydrase (enzyme/catalyst) to form carbonic acid (H_2CO_3). Without the catalyst, this change occurs very slowly. CO_2 is continually removed by respiratory ventilation and thereby kept at a steady state. The change in dissolved CO_2 in body fluids is proportional to pCO_2 in the gas phase.

Small animals are similar to humans with an open system for CO_2. The circulatory system and respiratory systems eliminate CO_2 at the rate it is produced and compensate when changes in $[H^+]$ occur. Increased amounts of CO_2 in the presence of a negative [SID] have a minimal effect on $[H^+]$. However, if increased CO_2 is present concurrently with positive [SID], the $[H^+]$ increases dramatically. This is demonstrated in the following equation:

$$[\text{SID}]+\left[H^+\right]-\left[HCO_3^-\right]-\left[A^-\right]-\left[CO_3^{2-}\right]-\left[OH^-\right]=0(\text{electrical neutrality}).$$

When circulating plasma $[H^+]$ changes occur due to changes in [SID], the respiratory rate will change to compensate and change the CO_2 level accordingly.

Compensation

According to strong ion theory, alterations involving [SID], pCO_2, or $[A_{TOT}]$ may occur in any one of these variables, resulting in compensatory changes in the other two. In cases of chronic hypercapnia, increases in $[HCO_3^-]$ and compensatory hypochloremia are noted. Traditional theory does not provide a definitive explanation as to why this occurs. However, Stewart's theory postulates that chronic hypercapnia stimulates a decrease in $[Cl^-]$ which in turn lowers [SID] and increases $[HCO_3^-]$, as HCO_3^- is considered to simply be a dependent variable. Patients experiencing hypocapnia however, have decreased pCO_2 and increased pH. After 24–48 hours, a reduction in $[HCO_3^-]$ is then noted. In addition, strong-ion weak-acid concentrations of albumin and phosphate will increase, without significantly changing the [SID]. This returns pH to normal with only minimal decreases in $[HCO_3^-]$. Changes in other variables, similar to those described above are seen if changes occur in any of these three variables. In turn, the other two will adjust to maintain pH.

Simplified approaches to strong ion?

There are three approaches to a simplified way of utilizing Stewart's theory of strong ions in clinical practice:
• Stewart–Figge methodology
• BE approach
• Constables simplified strong ion model.

Stewart–Figge methodology
Figge and others developed a mathematical approach in using strong ions to evaluate acid-base disorders. This methodology, however, has not been successfully tested in dogs or cats. The model utilizes protein-behavior based on human albumin and may not be accurate in the veterinary setting. These calculations, despite being termed "simplified", are generally not considered practical for daily use.

Base excess (BE) approach
In the traditional approach a negative BE is supportive of a metabolic acidosis. BE is a measurement of the buffer base, which is equivalent to the SID. BE values of less than −5 mmol/L are suggestive of increased unmeasured strong anions. Increased unmeasured strong anions would result in a decreased SID and subsequent acidosis. It must be considered that SID reflects just the serum levels, whereas BE is a reflection including the whole body and influence of hemoglobin. Yet there are a variety of equations that confirm that SID equates to this number for BE, so this may be a very simple way to approach incorporating

strong ion theory into clinical practice. However, this conclusion is based on human findings and in situations of normal protein levels. It is known that human albumin behaves differently on BE from that of dogs and cats. Further study would be necessary to confirm whether this approach was valuable in veterinary medicine and how altered protein and phosphate levels affected this approach.

Simplified strong ion model

SID, HCO_3^-, and A^- (protein weak acid buffers) are all considered in the equation $SID^+ = HCO_3^- + A^-$. This model takes into account that proteins act as strong ions, volatile buffer ions, or non-volatile buffer ions and assumes that every ionized entity in plasma can be classified in this manner (Morais & Constable 2006). This approach is still mechanistic and quantitative and does not eliminate the problems inherent in the Stewart model, namely the difficulty in accurately determining SID and the use of complex mathematics. Although these disadvantages limit the use of the Stewart model in the clinical setting, it is still preferred, owing to the ability to convey underlying mechanisms affecting a patient's acid-base status.

Strong ion gap (SIG)

SIG is often mentioned in light of the strong ion theory of acid-base. SIG is the difference between all unmeasured strong anions and all unmeasured strong cations, and is therefore another way that acid-base can be approached. A normal SIG is a positive number because there are more strong cations than strong anions. Unmeasured strong cations $[UC_{strong}^+]$ are ionized calcium and ionized magnesium. Unmeasured strong anions $[UA_{strong}^-]$ are ketones, lactate, and sulfate. Additionally strong ions must be measured to determine SIG, including sodium, potassium, and chloride. In this case the following formula is used:

$$SIG = \left[Na^+ \right] + \left[K^+ \right] - \left[Cl^- \right] = \left[UC_{strong}^+ \right] - \left[UA_{strong}^- \right]$$

Excess positively charged SIG is balanced by bicarbonate and non-volatile buffers $[A^-]$. Albumin is used to estimate $[A_{TOT}]$ (dogs with a normal plasma pH: $SIG_{simplified} = [alb] \times 4.9 - AG$; in cats: $SIG_{simplified} = [alb] \times 7.4 - AG$). When $SIG_{simplified}$ is <-5 mEq/L, increased unmeasured strong ions should be suspected and may be contributing to the change in pH.

If a patient is hyperphosphatemic, the AG must be adjusted with the following equation: $AG_{phosphate-adjusted} = AG + (2.52 - 0.58 \times [phosphate])$ prior to calculating the $SIG_{simplified}$. It is believed that the $SIG_{simplified}$ offers a more

Table 12.3 Strong ion effect on SID and acid-base status

↑or ↓	Ion Changed	Change to SID	A–B Change
↓	Chloride	Increased SID	Metabolic Alkalosis
↓	Sodium	Decreased SID	Metabolic Acidosis
↓	Albumin	Increased SID	Metabolic Alkalosis
↑	Chloride	Decreased SID	Metabolic Acidosis
↑	Phosphate	Decreased SID	Metabolic Acidosis
↑	Other (ketones, lactate)	Decreased SID	Metabolic Acidosis

accurate way to detect unmeasured strong ions than changes in AG alone. More testing is required to determine the accuracy of this theory and the equation in dogs and cats.

As previously noted, despite being "simplified", use of strong ion theory in daily practice is still far from simple. Stewart's approach may be most beneficial because it focuses on the 'whys' or reasons behind pH changes. Hydrogen, hydroxide, and bicarbonate are only dependent variables that occur due to these underlying causes. A major drawback with utilizing Steward's strong ion approach is that many calculations are required to understand it. In human medicine, computerized calculators have been created to perform strong ion assessment in clinical practice. On the other hand, small animal calculators utilizing gamblegrams are currently being developed by veterinarians in the critical care field (Lloyd 2004). Perhaps once they become common, this approach will gain popularity in its use. Nonetheless, there are insights that can be gained and applied daily in clinical practice by learning about and understanding the strong ion approach to acid-base. Putting into practice the effects of sodium and chloride (SID) on acid-base, as well as proteins and phosphorous (A_{TOT}), and knowing how increases or decreases may impact acid-base status, these conditions may be treated more effectively (Table 12.3). Doing so provides a more comprehensive approach to the critical care patient and provides greater insight into appropriate treatment and therapy options available.

References

Chawla, G. (2008). Water, strong ions, and weak ions. *Continuing Education in Anaesthesia, Critical Care & Pain* **8**(3): 108–12.

Constable P. D. (1999). Clinical assessment of acid-base status: Strong ion difference theory. *Veterinary Clinics of North America: Food animal practice* **15**(3): 447–71.

DiBartola, S. (ed.), (2006). Introduction to acid-base disorders. In: *Fluid, Electrolyte, and Acid-Base Disorders in Small Animal Practice*, 3rd ed. St Louis, MO: Saunders Elsevier: 229–49.

Grogono, A. (2011). Stewart's strong ion difference. In: *Acid-Base Tutorial*, http://www.acid-base.com/strongion.php.

Kellum, J. & Elbers, P. (2009). *Stewart's Textbook of Acid-Base*, 2nd ed. Amsterdam: Acidbase.org.

Kovacic, J. (2009). Acid-base disturbances. In: D. Silverstein & K. Hopper (eds), *Small Animal Critical Care Medicine*. St Louis, MO: Saunders Elsevier: 249–54.

Lloyd, P. (2004). Strong ion calculator: A practical bedside application of modern quantitative acid-base physiology. *Critical Care and Resuscitation* **6**: 285–94.

Morais, H. & Constable, P. (2006). Strong ion approach to acid-base disorders. In: S. DiBartola (ed.), *Fluid, Electrolyte, and Acid-Base Disorders in Small Animal Practice*, 3rd ed. St Louis, MO: Saunders Elsevier: 310–321.

Nickson, C. (2012). *Strong Ion Difference*, http://lifeinthefastlane.com/education/ccc/strong-ion-difference/.

Worthley, L. (1999). Strong ion difference: A new paradigm or new clothes for the acid-base emperor. *Critical Care and Resuscitation* **1**: 211–214.

CHAPTER 13

Companion Exotic Animal Electrolyte and Acid-Base

Jody Nugent-Deal, RVT, VTS (Anesthesia/Analgesia & Clinical Practice-Exotic Companion Animal) and Stephen Cital, RVT, RLAT, SRA

Companion exotic animals have become common household pets over the last few decades. Due to their popularity, advanced veterinary care is now in high demand. Compared to canine and feline patients, arterial and venous blood gas analysis and the evaluation of electrolyte values in most exotic animal species is still in its infancy. There are currently an estimated 10,000 species of birds, over 5,000 species of mammals, and at least 9,000 species of reptiles. Electrolyte and acid-base control is highly variable among the tens of thousands of different specially adapted species of animals throughout the world. Factors such as the phylum, genus, life-stage, metabolic rate, and environment are all contributing factors to the regulation and use of these physiologic processes. Common values for a majority of these species are unknown, due to a lack of published research. Those working with exotic animals often extrapolate from the current published data of similar species. This chapter of the text is designed to give an overview of the unique physiology and basic clinical principles involved with these homeostatic processes in exotic species. The authors have taken into account many of the specialized adaptations in exotic small mammals, birds, reptiles, amphibians and fish. It should be noted there are numerous interspecies anatomical and physiological evolutionary qualities giving each individual species their own adaptive edge. Species-specific research is highly encouraged, as discussing every species' particular physiology would be nearly impossible for this text.

Sample collection methods

Collection methods and sites will vary based on species, size of patient, and the amount of blood needed. Each species section will cover the more common means of intravenous and arterial access. Most exotic animals are prey species

Acid-Base and Electrolyte Handbook for Veterinary Technicians, First Edition.
Edited by Angela Randels-Thorp and David Liss.
© 2017 John Wiley & Sons, Inc. Published 2017 by John Wiley & Sons, Inc.
Companion website: www.wiley.com/go/liss/electrolytes

and/or have an increased fight or flight response. Causing extreme stress in an exotic animal can lead to death; therefore it is recommended that only experienced staff members handle, restrain, and collect blood for analysis. Sedation and/or general anesthesia should be considered in patients that require arterial cannulation and in those that are anxious. Sedating or anesthetizing a patient can help prevent iatrogenic trauma and large hematoma formation over the collection site. Anesthetic protocols and monitoring will vary by species. Only experienced veterinary practitioners should administer anesthetic drugs or perform general anesthesia. An exotic animal formulary should be consulted when necessary as these patients are unique and have different anesthetic requirements compared to dogs and cats.

Regardless of whether a venous or arterial sample is needed, blood obtained for analysis is generally collected into a 1 cc syringe heparinized with lithium heparin. A heparinized insulin syringe can also be used in very small patients. Blood should be analyzed within a few minutes of collection to ensure the most accurate results are obtained. Erroneous sodium results can occur with blood stored in heparin for longer periods of time. Blood samples can also be collected from indwelling catheters and are often a better option when serial samples are needed. Table 13.1 shows common intravenous and arterial catheterization sites in exotic animal patients.

Sample collection storage

Due to the size of most exotic animals, small blood volumes are generally collected for sampling. Microtainer® tubes are ideal because they are made for processing small volumes of blood. You can place as little of 0.1 cc of blood into the EDTA and heparin tubes. Placing small volumes of blood into the tubes commonly used for dogs and cats will cause dilution of the sample and skew the results.

EDTA can cause hemolysis in some reptilian and avian species, most commonly chelonians. The use of heparin will negate this, but may not be ideal if processing other blood samples. Lithium heparin can cause a blue-tinged staining to the cells and clumping of the thrombocytes and leukocytes, making interpretation of the CBC results more difficult. The authors suggest taking a blood sample via a clean syringe and first making a blood smear before placing the remaining blood into the EDTA and heparin or non-additive tubes (Bounous 2010).

Basic blood gas analysis of exotic species

Arterial blood gas monitoring is considered the "gold standard" method used to evaluate gas exchange and acid-base status in humans and canine/feline patients. Venous blood gas analysis is primarily used to assess values such as electrolytes

Table 13.1 Catheterization sites for common exotic animals

	Common vessel site(s)	Catheter size
Snakes	Jugular: must perform surgical cut-down – not common Tail: ventral aspect is the most common, potentially can place from the lateral aspect Carotid artery	26–20 g catheter – depends on size of patient
Lizards	Jugular and cephalic: must perform surgical cut-down – not common Tail: ventral aspect is the most common, potentially can place from the lateral aspect Carotid artery	26–20 g catheter – depends on size of the patient
Chelonians	Jugular: most common Tail: placed in the same manner as a lizard or snake Carotid artery	26–20 g catheter – depends on size of the patient
Rabbits	Cephalic, lateral saphenous and auricular veins Jugular: less common Auricular artery	26–20 g catheter – depends on size of the patient
Ferrets	Cephalic and lateral saphenous veins Jugular: less common Caudal tail artery	26–24 g catheter
Chinchilla/ Guinea pig	Cephalic and lateral saphenous Femoral artery	26–24 g catheter
Small rodents	Cephalic, lateral saphenous, tail Jugular: less common Femoral artery	26–24 g catheter
Birds	Medial metatarsal: medium to large birds Cutaneous ulnar and jugular veins: small to large birds Cutaneous ulnar artery: small to large birds	26–20 g catheter – depends on size of patient

and overall metabolic status. There are many different blood gas analyzers on the market today ranging from large, advanced tabletop machines to handheld bedside monitors such as an i-Stat®. Both varieties have advantages and disadvantages, but both provide similar data for interpretation. Analyzers should be chosen based on clinic need, staffing abilities, and budget. Because many exotic animal species are small, the machine chosen should be able to run a full panel on a minimal volume of blood.

Most blood gas analyzers provide values for pH, $PaCO_2$ (partial pressure of carbon dioxide), PaO_2 (partial pressure of oxygen), SaO_2 (oxygen saturation), and HCO_3^- (bicarbonate level). Other common values often include electrolytes, hemoglobin, base excess/deficit, and lactate.

The normal pH in birds ranges from 7.33 to 7.45; in mammals it is 7.35 to 7.45. The normal pH range in reptiles is likely similar based on known values. As

Table 13.2 The relationship between pCO_2 and pH when various metabolic disturbances are present

	pCO2	pH
Respiratory Acidosis	Increases	Decreases
Respiratory Alkalosis	Decreases	Increases
Metabolic Acidosis	Decreases	Decreases
Metabolic Alkalosis	Increases	Increases

with other species, values below the low end of the range indicate an acidosis and values above the high end of the range indicate an alkalosis; Table 13.2). While differences exist amongst species, the same basic rules for blood gas analysis still apply. The relationship between CO_2 and pH is inversely proportional. As the pH increases, the CO_2 decreases and as the pH decreases the CO_2 increases. Therefore as the CO_2 levels become elevated (primarily due to poor ventilation), the pH decreases, and the patient develops a respiratory acidosis. Conversely, as the CO_2 levels become decreased (primarily from hyperventilation, or cardiac shunting (reptiles)), the pH increases and the patient develops a respiratory alkalosis (Schumacher & Mans 2014).

Alternatives to blood gas analysis

Due to the lack of published reference ranges and the difficulty in sample collection across most exotic animal species, capnography can be used in lieu of blood gas analysis when necessary. A capnograph is an indirect measurement of arterial CO_2 and can be used to help assess ventilation in anesthetized and intubated patients. $ETCO_2$ correlates well with $PaCO_2$. $ETCO_2$ is the expired amount of carbon dioxide exhaled from the patient. Normal $ETCO_2$ levels range between 35 and 45 in most birds and mammals. In reptiles, it is common to see values around 20 mmHg (give or take) even though they should be in the same range as other animals.

In birds and mammals, patients are considered hypercapnic (too much CO_2) when $ETCO_2$ is greater than 45 mmHg. Increased values indicate inadequate ventilation, re-breathing of CO_2, or hypoventilation. Prolonged values reading above 60 mmHg can lead to hypoxemia. Hypoxemia predisposes patients to arrhythmias, myocardial depression, respiratory acidosis, and in rare cases, heart failure. In these cases, patients should be manually or mechanically ventilated to decrease $ETCO_2$. Hypoventilation can also indicate too deep of an anesthetic plane. Vitals and anesthetic depth should be assessed and adjusted as needed.

$ETCO_2$ values that are less than 35 mmHg can indicate hyperventilation. These patients are considered hypocapnic (not enough CO_2). Ventilation may also be required to help regulate erratic breathing patterns such as tachypnea. Hyperventilation can also indicate a light anesthetic plane or pain. This should be assessed and dealt with accordingly. Hypocapnia can also indicate other issues such as V/Q mismatch, decreased cardiac output, and esophageal intubation, extubation of the patient, kink or mucus plug in the tube, apnea, cardiac shunting of blood (reptiles), and hypothermia. Even though the above normal values used for birds and mammals do not apply to reptiles, the same signs and symptoms are still often valid.

In mammals, the measurement of $ETCO_2$ reads about 5–7 mmHg lower than actual $PaCO_2$. In birds, the opposite is true. The anatomy and physiology of the avian lung is quite different from that of mammals. Bird lungs create an efficient cross-current exchange system, which produces a higher concentration of CO_2 in expired gas compared to the actual arteries. This denotes that the $ETCO_2$ reading on the capnogram will be higher than the actual $PaCO_2$. In birds, it is estimated that the $ETCO_2$ reading will be about 5 mmHg higher than the $PaCO_2$ reading (Longley 2008).

Reptiles are vastly different compared to both mammals and birds. The anatomy and physiology varies greatly across species. All non-crocodilian hearts have three chambers consisting of two atria and one ventricle. The reptilian heart contains a pressure differential that exists between the chambers. This pressure differential ensures that oxygenated and pre-oxygenated blood do not mix together. Changes in pulmonary resistance allows for blood to either shunt from left to right (normal) or right to left (used during long periods of apnea often experienced with diving or when there is pulmonary pathology present). Shunting of blood from right to left bypasses the lungs and reduces systemic oxygen and heat loss. This often causes a ventilation/perfusion mismatch that is well tolerated by reptilian species. This is also likely the cause of decreased $ETCO_2$ measurements during anesthesia. Intra-cardiac shunting and various temperature gradients also lead to inaccurate interpretation of blood gases (Longley 2008).

Exotic small mammals

Respiratory system

The respiratory physiology of most mammals is very similar, as with arterial blood gas values. In general the smaller a mammal, the higher the metabolic rate becomes, which causes greater oxygen demand and requires greater oxygen delivery. Anatomical variances are few with only minor species differences in lung and thoracic compliance and bronchial and alveoli size. For information on mammalian respiratory physiology, please refer to Chapter 10. However, certain species—such as diving, burrowing, and hibernating animals—have adaptive traits to deal with their specialized lifestyles (Boggs, Kilgore, & Birchard 1984).

Smaller mammals, such as rodents and lagomorphs, have a high larynx within the oropharynx, making them obligate nasal breathers. To facilitate an increasing oxygen demand for quicker metabolism the animals have evolved high chest wall compliance, enabling them to expand their lungs better. They also have more alveoli of a thinner diameter to allow maximum oxygen exchange. Shorter airways and an increased respiratory rate also better increase oxygen demands. Higher metabolic rates increase body temperature, which prevents panting and loss of water (Helmer, Lewingtin, & Whiteside 2005).

Hibernation and torpor

Despite increased metabolic rates among species, hibernating or torpid species of animals have a significant drop in metabolic rate, lessening the burden of oxygen demand on energy reserves. A study comparing metabolic energy saved during hibernation in cold temperatures showed anywhere from 30 to 98.5% over normothermic basal-metabolic rates (Davenport 1992). However, the lack of water and cool to freezing temperatures can create other physiologic and biochemistry concerns. It is not fully understood how tissues can tolerate severe cold or how heart tissue can accommodate such low rates and temperatures without damage. One example comes from hibernation research performed on ground squirrels whose heart rate at normal temperatures is 240 beats per minute. During hibernation in temperatures as low as 2–7 °C, a squirrel's heart rate drops to 3–4 beats per minute with decreased cardiac output, but with normal aortic pressure.

Acidosis is another common event seen in hibernating animals. Respiratory rates can drop extremely low (1–2 breaths per minute), with an increase in pCO_2 levels and drop in pH. The general pH depression does help with energy saving, due to metabolic inhibition. However, pH levels will stay near or at normal ranges at the expense of proton pumping of energy reserves allowing for normal enzyme function.

In bears body temperatures may not drop as dramatically compared to small mammal species. Interestingly bears do not void urine or defecate during hibernation. Although small amounts of urine are still created it is stored in the urinary bladder until reemergence. The bladder does act as a site of water and nitrogen reabsorption (Davenport 1992).

Renal function and osmoregulation

Mammalian renal function is generally very similar across the thousands of different species with common variances in shape, location, and size. A species' environment and diet will also play a role on the limited, but notable, physiology. Desert species will need to be able to reabsorb and concentrate urine, while others will need to be able to handle increased water intake, high protein, and salty diets.

Rabbit kidneys are particularly interesting considering their primitive design and physiology compared to other mammals. Lagomorph species have glomeruli that are not active all at once, but can be utilized with an increase in water intake. Because rabbits utilize bacterial fermentation, they can have high levels of bicarbonate, making them more prone to alkalosis. Consequently, this leads to more alkaline urine that may appear milky, due to calcium carbonate excretion. Compared to other mammalian species, rabbit kidneys are excellent at excreting dietary calcium. Typically, most mammals will only excrete ~2% of calcium via urine and the rest through bile, while rabbits will excrete ~60% via urine. Lacking normal mammalian ammonium buffering, rabbits are more susceptible to acid loads.

Osmoregulation is predominately controlled by drinking and diet. Certain desert species of rodents can create metabolic water in exceptionally dry periods, but will eventually need to find sources of drinking water or food where water can be absorbed during digestion.

Electrolyte and acid-base

Electrolyte and acid-base changes in rodents, primates, and lagomorphs, along with a whole host of more exotic mammal species, are the same as described in typical small animal practice via serum or plasma. A species environment and diet will be the major contributing factors to the variances seen with electrolyte physiology, such as desert species verses saltwater aquatic species of mammals (Bradshaw, Morris, & Bradshaw 2001).

Collection sites

There are several sites that can be used for blood collection in exotic small mammals. Collection sites will vary by species as well as the preference and skill of the phlebotomist. Average circulating blood volume in the exotic small mammal ranges between 6 and 7%. No more than 10% of the total circulating blood volume should be taken from a healthy patient (Lennox & Bauck 2012). For example, a 1 kg rabbit has a circulating blood volume of approximately 60 cc. In a healthy patient, a total volume of 6 cc can be taken safely for sampling (although other potential blood loss needs to be taken into account).

Ferrets

Venipuncture sites in the ferret include the cephalic, lateral saphenous, jugular, and cranial vena cava vessels. Blood can be obtained from the peripheral vessels and the jugular vein in a similar manner as in a dog (note that the skin is thick and the jugular vessel is more lateral compared to that of a dog or cat). Syringe and needle size will vary, but in general a 1 cc syringe with a 25-gauge needle attached is used for peripheral vessels while a 1 or 3 cc syringe with a 25- or 22-gauge needle attached is used for the jugular vein. The cranial vena cava is generally the quickest method that may yield the largest amount of blood. If the cranial vena cava is used, the animal must be placed under general anesthesia or heavy sedation before the sample is collected. A 25-gauge needle attached to a 1 or 3 cc syringe is used for this venipuncture site. The patient is placed in dorsal recumbency with the front legs pulled down next to the body and the head and neck extended. The needle should be aimed toward the opposite hind limb and is then inserted at a 45-degree angle into the thoracic inlet. The landmarks used to find the cannulation site include the manubrium and the first rib. This is the same technique used in other exotic small mammals. Collection of arterial blood samples can be difficult in ferrets. The femoral artery is easy to palpate and blood is collected in the same manner as a dog. The caudal tail artery is another option but, in the authors' opinion, more difficult, due to the size of the vessel. Collection at this site requires a steady hand. A heparinized insulin or 1 cc syringe attached to a 27-gauge needle is used for cannulation. The caudal tail artery runs on midline along the ventral aspect of the tail. Samples are obtained by inserting the syringe and needle at approximately a 30- to 45-degree angle. Slight negative pressure should be placed on the syringe once the needle penetrates the skin. The needle and syringe is slowly advanced until the artery is cannulated and blood enters into the hub. If the needle touches bone, it has been advanced too far. The needle should be backed out slowly, keeping slight negative pressure on the syringe until blood fills the hub. Arterial cannulation generally requires sedation.

Chinchillas
Venipuncture sites in the chinchilla include the cephalic, lateral saphenous, and jugular veins. The peripheral vessels do not generally yield enough blood for most diagnostic samples; therefore the jugular vein is most often the vessel of choice for obtaining blood. Performing jugular venipuncture on a chinchilla is similar to that on a cat. It is important that those restraining are aware of fur-slip. Chinchillas being prey species have the ability to lose large sections of fur when grabbed. This is an adaptation to help escape predation. A 27- or 25-gauge needle attached to a 1 cc syringe is most commonly used for blood collection. Animals that are uncooperative may need light sedation to obtain the sample. Arterial sampling is difficult in the chinchilla, due to their small size. The femoral artery is most often cannulated when an arterial blood sample is needed. This is done using the same technique in canine patients.

Rabbits
Venipuncture sites in the rabbit are very similar to those used in dogs and include the cephalic, lateral saphenous, auricular, and jugular veins. The jugular veins can be difficult to obtain blood from in rabbits that have large dewlaps or those that are grossly obese. Performing jugular venipuncture on rabbits is done in the same manner as canine and feline patients. The cephalic and auricular vessels are generally small and may not yield enough blood for diagnostic sampling. The lateral saphenous veins are usually the quickest and easiest sites for sampling. Obtaining blood from the lateral saphenous in a rabbit is accomplished in the

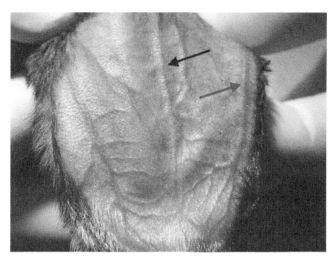

Figure 13.1 The pinna of the rabbit is quite vascular. The blue arrow is pointing to the marginal auricular vein while the black arrow is pointing to the auricular artery.

same manner as in a dog. A 1 cc syringe with a 27- or 25-gauge needle should be used. Proper restraint is a must. The peripheral vessels are extremely friable and blow easily.

Obtaining arterial blood samples in rabbits is generally quite easy. The median auricular artery is large and runs down the middle of the pinna (Figure 13.1). The auricular artery may spasm when either a needle or catheter is inserted into the vessel. Placing a thin layer of local anesthetic cream over the skin and covering the artery with a semi-occlusive bandage for 20 minutes can help lessen the possibility of occurrence (Figure 13.2). Drawing blood from the auricular artery is best accomplished by having an assistant gently restrain the patient while the phlebotomist stabilizes the pinna with one hand and obtains the sample using a 1 cc syringe with a 27-gauge attached with the other hand. Most rabbits will not need sedation for sample collection. The pinna is hard to bandage; therefore pressure should be applied to the vessel by hand to prevent hematoma formation. Although rare, the pinna can slough, due to large hematoma formation after either venous or arterial blood draws. The femoral artery can also be used for sample collection, but this is generally not necessary, because the auricular artery is almost 100% successful.

Guinea pigs

The peripheral vessels as well as the jugular vein can be used to obtain blood samples from the guinea pig. The needle and syringe size as well as the positioning are the same for the chinchilla. The cephalic vein is usually too small to obtain a substantial sample, but the lateral saphenous vein can often be used to obtain about 1 cc of blood or less. Guinea pigs have very stocky, short necks,

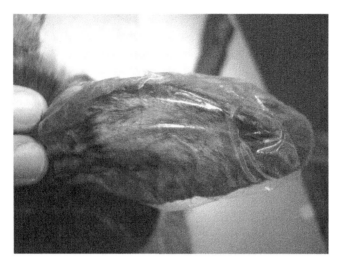

Figure 13.2 The auricular artery is used for blood gas sampling in exotic mammals such as rabbits. The artery is numbed prior to sampling by applying a thin layer of local anesthetic cream to the surface and then covering it with a semi-occlusive bandage.

making it difficult to use the jugular vessels for sample collection. In the authors' opinion, if the lateral saphenous is not an option, the second best vessel to obtain a blood sample from is the femoral vein. Obtaining blood from the femoral vein is generally the quickest method that yields the largest amount of blood. The sample can be taken once the patient is properly anesthetized. The patient is anesthetized to minimize the chance of lacerating the large femoral vessels. To obtain the blood sample, first palpate the pulse of the femoral artery in the inguinal area. The nipple can be used as a landmark to help find the pulse. Because the artery and the vein run alongside each other, the arterial pulse is used to help pinpoint the location of the vein. Once the artery is palpated, the needle (it is best to use a 1 cc tuberculin syringe with a 25- or 22-gauge needle) should be inserted at a 45-degree angle into the skin. This venipuncture site is a blind stick. Since the vessel cannot be visualized, it is important to place slight negative pressure on the syringe as soon as the needle enters the skin. Having negative pressure on the syringe is helpful for the phlebotomist because blood will enter the syringe once the needle is properly placed into the vessel. Without negative pressure on the syringe, it is very easy to unknowingly go through the vessel. Once the blood sample has been obtained, the needle can be removed and the thumb or a finger is placed over the insertion site to hold off the vessel.

Blood can also be obtained from the cranial vena cava (same procedure as used in a ferret), but this does not come without potential risk of traumatic bleeding into the thoracic cavity or pericardial sac. If the cranial vena cava is chosen as the venipuncture site, the animal must be under general anesthesia while obtaining the blood sample. A struggling patient can greatly increase the risk of lacerating the vena cava during sample collection; therefore this venipuncture site should never be used when an animal is awake. The same is true for chinchillas. It can be used in chinchillas and other small rodents, but it does not come without risk.

Arterial blood collection can be challenging in guinea pigs. The only viable option is the femoral artery. The same procedure discussed for femoral venipuncture applies to the collection of blood from the femoral artery. Because this is a blind stick, it can be hard to differentiate between cannulation of the vein or artery. Arterial blood will often fill the syringe much faster than venous blood. Normal arterial blood is a brighter red color, and running an arterial blood gas will confirm the origins of its collection.

Rodents

Blood collection from small rodents—such as mice, rats, and hamsters—is challenging. The peripheral veins as well as the jugular vein can be used but, again, these vessels are small and it is hard to obtain sample sizes large enough to run a variety of diagnostic samples. In rats and mice, the lateral tail veins can be used to obtain small amounts of blood. The vessels are usually superficial and can easily be seen (unless the animal is very debilitated or obese). This can be accomplished by either using an insulin syringe or 1 cc syringe with 27-gauge needle. A 27- or 25-gauge needle can also be placed into the vessel. Once there is blood in the hub of the needle, a hematocrit tube can be used to collect the blood (Figure 13.3).

Using the femoral vein to obtain a blood sample is generally the quickest method that will yield the largest volume of blood (Figure 13.4). The same method described in guinea pigs is also used with hamsters, mice, and rats,

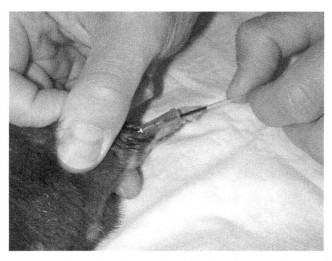

Figure 13.3 Venipuncture in small rodents can be difficult. To help keep the vessel from collapsing, a small-gauge needle can be inserted into the vessel and blood can be collected using several hematocrit tubes.

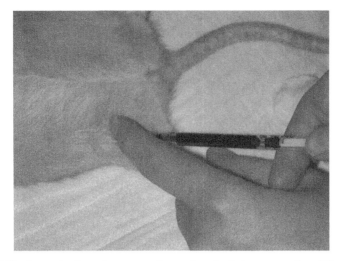

Figure 13.4 The femoral vein and artery can be used to obtain larger samples of blood from small rodents. A 27- or 25-gauge needle attached to a 1 cc syringe works well for sample collection.

although a 27- or 25-gauge needle attached to a 1 cc syringe is generally used. Arterial samples can be obtained from the femoral artery using the technique described in the guinea pig section.

Birds

Respiratory system

Birds have an increased metabolism compared to mammals of a similar size, meaning they have increased oxygen demands. The avian respiratory system consists of non-expandable parabronchial lungs and an average of nine air sacs, while lacking a diaphragm. Air sacs in avian species are poorly vascularized and do not participate in gas exchange, but rather act as bellows to the functional lung tissue. The blood gas barrier of birds is 2.5 times thinner than mammals and is supported externally (West 2009). Birds also have diverticula, which are air sac like pouches, into bones such as the humerus, femur, cervical vertebrae, sternum ribs, pelvis, and pectoral girdle. Air capillaries (equivalent to mammalian alveoli) are more numerous in birds. The capillaries are so thin the larger avian erythrocytes must line up to pass through. In species that fly at high altitudes the Hb has a higher oxygen affinity to deal with lower oxygen levels. Blood gas barriers depend on species and are thinner in flying birds vs. terrestrial species. Birds also have a highly variable and sometimes long tracheal anatomy. An avian breath is a two-part cycle for complete gas exchange. This is technically more advantageous, resulting in a much slower respiratory rate than that of similar sized mammals. Air from the first inspiration enters the trachea and moves into the primary bronchus and neopulmonic region. The air then moves to the caudal air sacs. There also may be some movement of air into the paleopulmonic regions, where gas exchange can occur. Some species, like emus and penguins, only have paleopulmonic parabronchial tissue. With the first expiration, the air in the caudal air sacs largely moves to the paleopulmonic region with about 12% loss escaping out the trachea through bidirectional neopulmonic regions.

With the second inspiration, the remaining air from the paleopulmonic regions moves into the cranial air sacs. With the second expiration, the air moves from the cranial air sacs out through the bronchi and lastly through the trachea. Again, about another 12% of air escapes in this cycle through the neopulmonic regions out the trachea without full gas exchange.

Renal function and osmoregulation

The role of avian kidneys is like that of other species, filtering water and waste substances from blood, to eventually be voided from the body. Avian kidneys also play an important role in conserving water and reabsorbing needed substances. The avian kidney is divided into lobules, each containing a cortex and medulla with dual afferent blood supply. Avian kidneys have more medullary nephrons to concentrate urine.

The functional unit of the kidney is the nephron, of which birds have two kinds. The reptilian-type, with no loops of Henle, is located in the cortex, while a more mammalian-type with long or intermediate length loops is located in the medulla. Only a small percentage of nephrons (<25%) contain a loop of Henle. Avian urine is semi-solid, consisting of urates (a white creamy precipitate) and supernatant fluid (urine). Glomerular filtration is responsible for urine production and 90% is reabsorbed by the tubules. Lacking urinary bladders, urine and urates meet at the cloaca and proceed by retro-peristalsis into the colon where further water absorption takes place.

Osmoregulation occurs by pure water, nectar, or succulent food intake. Species that live in arid conditions can create metabolic water with scant urine production. Birds in arid conditions excrete 55% water in their excrement compared to non-arid-living birds with 75–90% water excretion. Dehydration can lead to irreversible gout. Birds also conserve water by cooling warm air as it passes through their nares. Studies have shown birds are effective at cooling themselves by panting via evaporative cooling with minimal changes to acid-base and CO_2 levels. Dead space created by avian air sacs plays an important role in acid-base regulation during panting (Long 1981; Marder & Arad 1989). High-altitude flyers or migratory birds that can fly and fast for 72 hr don't suffer water loss due to the elevation (cooler air) and metabolic water production from fat in the liver.

Nasal glands exist in some species of birds that live in freshwater-deprived environments. Salt glands are distinct from lacrimal or Harderian glands. Marine species are particularly well developed to allow the animal to drink seawater and excrete the salt through a sneeze. The glands are similar to renal tissue with countercurrent blood flow (Campbell 2004a; Helmer & Whiteside 2005a).

Avian species that survive by nectar diets, like the hummingbird, have special kidney and osmoregulatory mechanisms to deal with large amounts of water containing only scant amounts of protein and electrolytes with high osmotic concentrations (McWhorter & Del Rio 1999).

Birds can also conserve water by cooling warm air through their nares and have decreased water waste in their excrement compared to birds in water-rich environments.

Electrolyte and acid-base

The primary active osmotic electrolyte in birds is sodium. Acquired from the bird's diet, sodium is absorbed via the gastrointestinal (GI) tract and then sent to the kidneys for dispersal or excretion. In certain species salt glands near the nares help alleviate surplus sodium. It has been documented that birds with salt glands can expel 60–88% of excess sodium via these glands instead of renal excretion. Hyponatremia (<130 mEq/L) and hypernatremia (>160 mEq/L) disorders have the same etiologies as in mammal species. However, sea birds, when kept in captivity and given freshwater, can get atrophy of the salt glands and become hypernatremic as a result. Hypernatremia is greater in species that lack salt glands. Imbalanced salt intakes and dehydration can contribute to hypernatremia.

Chloride is the highest concentrated anion in the extracellular fluid. Imbalances are rarely reported. The typical normal range of chloride for many avian species is between 100 and 120 mEq/L. Excessive chloride has been associated with poor food intake and can partially inhibit anhydrase, which will have a direct impact on eggshell formation. Hypochloremia is associated with metabolic alkalosis like that in mammals.

Potassium is the most abundant intracellular cation and disturbances echo mammalian disorders. Typical potassium levels are between 2.0 and 4.0 mEq/L. Careful treatments with fluid support to either decrease or increase potassium levels with supplementation are recommended in birds when clinically necessary.

Calcium and phosphorus balance also echoes mammals. One major difference with avian species is in egg-laying females, which will have increased blood calcium levels.

Acid-base balance in birds is very similar to that in mammalian species with a normal pH range of 7.33–7.45. Other studies have shown birds, depending on temperature, have slightly alkaline pH and lower pCO_2 (Long 1981). In general practice acid-base disorders are rarely corrected otherwise.

Because of their unique respiratory system, respiratory-related imbalances in birds can change positively and negatively rather quickly, and corrected via manual or mechanical ventilation likewise in anesthetized birds. Roughly 99% or greater of daily acid excretion is in the form of CO_2 via respiration. The bicarbonate and carbonic acid buffering system is pivotal in the acid-base balance of birds, due to their more effective elimination of CO_2. Renal involvement with acid-base balance by recuperation of buffers, with excretion of acid, is also highly dependent on temperature, increasing filtration rates as core temperature rises. Other non-bicarbonate buffering mechanisms are likely to play a role in avian acid-base regulation like in mammals, primarily by proteins (Campbell 2004a; Helmer & Whiteside 2005a; Long 1981).

Collection sites

Obtaining blood from the avian patient can be challenging, but being consistently successful is an important and valuable skill to possess. Collection sites in birds include the jugular, cutaneous ulnar (basilic vein) and medial metatarsal veins and the cutaneous ulnar (basilic) artery. The medial metatarsal veins are generally the most commonly used vessels for obtaining blood in medium and large birds (Figure 13.5). The jugular vein is often used when large samples of blood are needed or in very small species, such as finches, canaries, and cockatiels. The right jugular vein is usually larger in most species of birds and is more often chosen over the left jugular vein (Figure 13.6 and Figure 13.7). The cutaneous ulnar vein can be used in larger species of birds, but it is hard to bandage and often forms a large hematoma if poor hemostasis occurs or if the bird flaps its wing. The cutaneous ulnar artery is most commonly cannulated for blood gas sample collection. Arterial cannulation can be painful in any species and may bleed heavily, leading to large hematoma formation. It is suggested that pressure is placed over the collection site for at least 5 minutes.

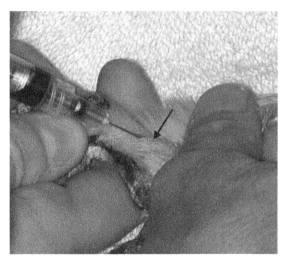

Figure 13.5 The black arrow is pointing to the medial metatarsal vein in an avian patient. The person restraining the bird holds off the vessel by placing a finger or thumb across the leg similar to what is done in a canine or feline patient. The syringe and needle size used will be based on the size of the patient. In general a 1 or 3 cc syringe attached to a 27- or 25-gauge needle is used for sample collection.

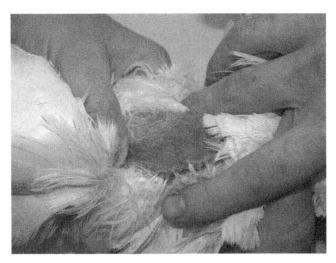

Figure 13.6 The jugular vein can be used for sample collection in most species of birds. The right jugular vein is often larger than the left, but either vessel can be cannulated.

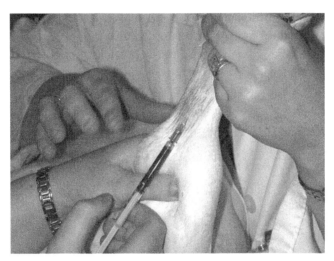

Figure 13.7 The syringe and needle size used will be based on the size of the patient. In general a 1 or 3 cc syringe attached to a 27- or 25-gauge needle is used for sample collection.

How much blood can you safely take from a small bird such as a 1 kg macaw? Blood volume is often not thought of when taking a blood sample from most dogs and cats, but it is something you *must* consider when drawing blood from most avian patients. Circulating blood volume is approximately 10% of the body weight. Approximately 1% of the body weight in blood can be taken for sampling (Bounous 2010). For example, a 1 kg macaw has a total of 100 cc of circulating blood. Of the 100 cc, 10 cc blood can be safely taken from a healthy patient. It is suggested that only half of the amount of blood is taken from a sick patient. Surgical blood loss and loss from a recent trauma should be taken into account prior to sampling.

Reptiles

Respiratory system

The reptilian respiratory anatomy and physiology are very primitive. In general reptilian pulmonary structures are simple sacs with invaginations called faveoli to increase the surface area. Faveoli are equivalent to alveoli in mammals. Reptiles, with the exception of crocodilian species, lack a diaphragm. The lung volume in reptiles is quite large but the "working' surface area is small respectively. They also lack a true thorax and abdomen, thus the entire trunk of the body is referred to as the coelom. Reptiles are prone to respiratory infections due to their primitive mucociliary apparatus making it difficult to clear debris from the airway.

Most snakes have only one functional unicameral lung on the right side, meaning that there is one sac-like structure. The left side is vestigial or absent. Boidae are the exception: both the left and right lungs are functional.

Lizard lungs also vary by species. Some lizard species are unicameral, most common in skinks. Other species such as chameleons have paucicameral lungs, meaning they are still very sac-like but there are also a few simple divisions within the lungs. The last type of lung found in lizards is multicameral. The multicameral lung is found in iguana species. This type of lung has multiple chambers (Campbell 2004b).

Chelonian species have paired multicameral lungs. Due to the presence of the shell and lack of a true diaphragm, movement of the legs and head/neck aid in respiration. When chelonian species retract into their shells they cannot move their pectoral girdle and must breath hold. When these species are anesthetized, this movement ceases and apnea occurs. This is the main reason for intermittent positive pressure ventilation (IPPV) under anesthesia. Small tidal volumes can be exchanged by moving the hind legs in and out of the shell when anesthetized in a pumping fashion. Some chelonian species have cutaneous gas exchange through their skin, shell, pharyngeal mucosa, and/or cloacal bursae. This only occurs in some soft-shelled aquatic species.

Anaerobic metabolism is less efficient than aerobic metabolism but is common among reptiles, most commonly in chelonians species. Anaerobic metabolism is used for high-velocity activity and diving, with highly draining effects on energy reserves. During anaerobic activity, glycogen in the muscle is quickly converted into lactate, which takes longer to eliminate in reptiles, due to their overall slower metabolism. Reptiles can tolerate remarkably high levels of lactate compared to mammals with chelonians species having the highest levels recorded in blood chemistry research. Chelonians also have the highest bicarbonate levels of all vertebrates, which will help buffer lactic acid accumulation during anaerobic periods. Increases in lactate will drop the blood pH levels, decreasing oxygen affinity of Hb (Bohr effect), delaying oxygen transport, and further increasing anaerobic demand. Circulation can be shunted based on pulmonary resistance.

During peak respiratory activity, pulmonary resistance is low so deoxygenated blood flows through the pulmonary arch to the lungs while oxygenated blood flow systemically (Campbell 2004b; Helmer & Whiteside 2005b).

In mammals, acid-base balance and pCO_2 are essential in controlling respiration. Reptiles, on the other hand, are tolerant of hypoxia and extreme acid-base changes with temperature being the biggest factor of tolerability. Rising temperature increases oxygen demand, thus increasing tidal volumes of reptiles. High oxygen tension also decreases the respiratory rate, which can make anesthesia challenging since most hospitals only have 100% oxygen.

Reptiles are ectotherms, meaning their temperature is dependent on the surrounding temperature. A more appropriate term for many reptile species is poikilotherm. This is a more fitting term, since many reptiles often go through more variable core body temperature changes throughout the day. Some ectotherms can remain at a stable temperature depending on their environmental temperature fluctuations. There are species of boas and sea turtles that have brown fat which can be used to create metabolic heat, similar to mammals. Reptiles can heat up quicker than cool down. Blood shunting (quick right to left cardiac shunt) allows for bypassing evaporative effects/cooling from the lungs, conserving water, and thereby slowing cooling. This also has dramatic effects on blood gas values.

During hibernation the reptile seeks a moist den and prevention from freezing. Oxygen tension is not a concern as low metabolic rates and anaerobic metabolism make them tolerant to hypoxia. Fat in the liver, coelom, and tail provide energy that will be needed for reemerging. Aquatic hibernators will swim and rest at the bottom of ponds or lakes where water will not freeze where they switch to mostly anaerobic hibernation, while some species breathe dissolved oxygen in the water through cutaneous respiration.

Estivation in reptiles occurs in species that live in extremely dry terrain. Turtles species will bury themselves until moisture or cooler temperature triggers reemergence. Weight loss (no more than 10%) is expected from water and electrolyte loss during estivation (Campbell 2004b; Helmer & Whiteside 2005b).

Renal function and osmoregulation

Reptile kidneys are located in the caudal region of the coelom. Chelonian species have symmetrically placed kidneys, whereas some species of lizards have fused kidneys at midline. Formed from the posterior embryo, they are termed metanephric and excrete excess water, nitrogenous wastes like other species. They lack loops of Henle, meaning they cannot concentrate urine beyond the osmotic values of blood plasma. Reptile kidneys also lack a renal pelvis and pyramids. In male snakes and lizards the terminal segment has evolved into a sexual segment. Only a handful of reptile species have a urinary bladder. Species with urinary bladders drain urine into the cloaca, where it then enters the urinary bladder. Chelonians and species of lizards can use the bladder as a water reservoir or salt storage and for buoyancy. Species lacking a urinary bladder drain urine into the cloaca, where it is then pushed into the distal colon for final water absorption.

Aquatic reptiles excrete ammonia and urea with relatively small amounts of uric acid, as water is not crucial. Terrestrial species needing to conserve water excrete uric acid, which precipitates from solution in the bladder or cloaca, forming pasty white urates. Urate composition is heavy in either sodium (Na^+) or potassium (K^+) salts, depending on diet. Uric acid excretion is advantageous as it is insoluble and doesn't require much water to pass. While not in the animal's favor, uric acid is excreted through the kidney tubules using water to pass the solute through, even in times of suboptimal hydration. If an animal is extremely dehydrated or suffers from renal disease, this can quickly cause gout in the joints and visceral organs. Dietary gout can occur when herbivores are fed animal proteins, causing excess uric acid production and hyperuricemia. Nearly 60% of renal function must be lost before there is a significant rise in plasma uric acid, making it a less sensitive diagnostic indicator. Uric acid can also be higher post feeding in carnivorous reptile species, making fasting important for sample collection.

Reptile mass is generally 70% water with osmolarity varying greatly among the numerous species, adapted to each species' diet, environment, and lifestyle. Water intake is either by oral consumption, cutaneous absorption through less keratinized portion of their skin or between scales, or cloacal absorption. Tropical species of reptiles require an increased consumption of water compared to adapted desert species. The lowest osmolarity is seen in freshwater chelonian species and the highest in desert chelonian species (Campbell 2004b; Helmer & Whiteside 2005b).

Electrolyte and acid-base

Similar to mammalian physiology, the most prominent osmotic regulatory components of the blood plasma are sodium, chloride, and bicarbonate. However, osmolarity in reptiles is much less regulated compared to mammals, allowing for much greater variations and tolerability in regards to a species environment. Aquatic species' osmolarity will depend on the surrounding water concentrates, whereas terrestrial species' osmolarity will depend on the animal's hydration and is usually higher. Tolerability to what would be considered detrimental in mammals, such as an Na well over 170 mEq/L, might have little presenting clinical abnormalities in reptiles on physical exam. In fact, sodium contributes to about 90% of reptilian cations. Typical normal ranges of sodium in the reptile are between 120 and 170 mEq/L. See Table 13.3 for summary of electrolyte normal ranges relevant within the scope of this chapter. The more common reasons for hyponatremia in replies include diarrhea, kidney disease, salt gland disorders, and over-hydration.

Dehydration is the most common reason for hypernatremia, followed by increased dietary salts.

Table 13.3 Normal electrolyte ranges for common exotic animal (Source: Adapted from Carpenter 2013)

	Na$^+$	K$^+$	Cl$^-$	BG
Ferret	146–160	4.3–5.3	102–121	63–134
Rabbit	138–155	3.7–6.8	92–112	75–150
Chinchilla	142–166	3.3–5.7	108–129	109–193
Guinea pig	146–152	6.8–8.9	98–115	60–125
Rat	135–155	5.9	No value	50–135
African grey	134–152	2.6–4.2	No value	190–350
Boa	130–152	3.0–5.7	No value	10–60
Bearded dragon	145–167	2.6–5.0	111–141	149–253
Dessert tortoise	130–157	3.5–3.9	109–112	69–82
Koi	112–141	2.7–4.3	No value	22–65

Electrolytes such as potassium are well regulated in reptile species with little variability among species. Herbivorous species of reptiles consume relatively high levels of K$^+$ in their diets. Severe alkalosis and imbalanced diets have been associated with hypokalemia, where hyperkalemia can be seen with secretion issues either by the kidneys or salt glands. Sodium from the animal's diet is mainly absorbed via the GI tract and stored or sent to the kidneys. Excesses are excreted in their urine, while other excess physiologic salts can be excreted and sneezed out by nasal salt glands. See Table 13.4 for summary of causes of electrolyte abnormalities relevant within the scope of this chapter.

Clinically, chloride-related abnormalities are less common in reptiles and of less concern compared to mammals. Plasma concentrations of chloride in certain species, like crocodilians, can drop to near zero after feeding with compensatory factors increasing levels back to normal within short periods of time. Over-hydration can also lead to hypochloremia in non-feeding reptiles, while hyper-chloremia is suggestive of renal tubular disease or dehydration. Salt gland function can play a role in any reptilian electrolyte imbalance. Chloride with bicarbonate contributes about 80–90% of reptilian anions. Average reptilian chloride levels are 100–130 mEq/L (Dessauer 1970; Carpenter, Klaphake, & Gibbons 2014).

Calcium (Ca$^+$) and phosphorus (Phos) balance is key in reptiles. A total of 99% of Ca$^+$ is in the bones and must be maintained in the blood plasma as well for normal neuromuscular function. Calcium metabolism is regulated by para-thyroid hormone (PTH), activated vitamin D$_3$, and calcitonin. Calcitonin is still not fully understood in the reptile, but experts suggest it may be vital for antago-nizing PTH. When ionized Ca$^+$ drops, PTH increases and mobilizes Ca$^+$ from the bones. Drops in Ca$^+$ activate vitamin D$_3$ to increase GI absorption for supplemen-tation of Ca$^+$ and Phos. Reabsorption from the kidneys is also triggered with low Ca$^+$ levels. Metabolic bone disease occurs when there is insufficient Ca$^+$ in the diet.

Table 13.4 Common causes of electrolyte abnormalities (Source: Adapted from Harr 2006)

Calcium – Increased	• Reproductive
	• Hypervitaminosis D
	• Primary hyperparathyroidism
	• Renal Secondary hyperparathyroidism
	• Nutritional secondary hyperparathyroidism
	• Neoplasia
	• Osteomyelitis
Calcium – Decreased	• Nutritional
	• Chronic egg laying
	• Hypomagnesemia
	• Hypoparathyroidism
	• Pancreatitis
	• Malabsorption
	• Alkalosis
Chloride – Increased	• Dehydration
	• Metabolic Acidosis
Chloride – Decreased	• Vomiting
	• Metabolic alkalosis
Glucose – Increased	• Endocrine
	• Pancreatitis
	• Stress
	• Drugs
Glucose – Decreased	• Liver failure
	• Starvation
	• Neoplasia
	• Septicemia
Potassium – Increased	• Renal failure
	• Diabetic ketoacidosis
	• Severe tissue damage
	• Dehydration
	• Drugs
Potassium – Decreased	• Alkalosis
	• Drugs
	• GI loses
	• Chronic renal disease
Sodium – Increased	• Vomiting
	• Intestinal fluid loss
	• Renal failure
	• Dehydration
Sodium – Decreased	• Diabetes mellitus
	• Vomiting
	• Burns
	• Chronic effusion
	• Chronic renal failure

Ratios of Ca^+/Phos are ideally 2:1; however, high-protein diets have an inverse Ca^+/Phos ratio. Herbivore diets are low on Ca^+/Phos. Feeding reptiles prey with developed bones can alleviate dietary deficiencies (Campbell 2004b; Helmer & Whiteside 2005b).

Extreme acid-base variations are another remarkable adaptation of reptiles. Reptiles can have fluctuations that would be considered inconsistent with life in mammals. Blood samples in estuarine crocodiles collected immediately after capture had pH levels as low as 6.6. Loggerhead sea turtles also had sharp decreases in pH and bicarbonate with a dramatic increase in lactate after capture (Harms et al. 2003). Feeding crocodilian data have revealed alkalosis with concurrent hypochloremia and an increase in bicarbonate that eventually corrects itself after feeding. This effect was not seen in Savannah monitor lizards or python species, showing the highly variable acid-base regulatory process among species during postprandial alkaline tides in carnivorous reptilian species (Hartzler et al. 2006). Generally, reptile pH samples collected while at rest should be around 7.4–7.7. A machine calibrated to the animal's core body temperature is the only effective way to accurately assess reptilian blood samples. Increases in temperature are associated with dropping the pH. It is suggested that pH is regulated tightly, similar to mammals to within 0.2 pH units under normal species-optimal conditions (Harms et al. 2003). Chelonian species tend to be alkaline, averaging around 7.8 consistently. This adaptation could be part of their secret to long periods of anoxia and lactic acidosis in diving species, where pH levels may drop to 6.8 with an oxygen tension approaching zero. The oxygen disassociation curve for reptilian Hb, like mammals, will shift to the left as pH increases.

It is suspected that bicarbonate and carbonic acid are key factors in buffering blood after rapid CO_2 elimination during aerobic respiration (Dessauer 1970; Gibbons 2014).

Collection sites
Lizards
Blood collection sites will vary based on the species, size of the patient, and preference of the phlebotomist. Average circulating blood volume is approximately 5–8% of the body weight. No more than 10% of the total circulating blood volume should be taken from a healthy patient (Bounous 2010). For example, a 1 kg lizard has a circulating blood volume of approximately 50 cc. In a healthy patient, a total volume of 5 cc can be taken safely for sampling (although other potential blood loss needs to be taken into account).

The cephalic, jugular, and ventral abdominal vessels can be used to obtain a blood sample from various species of lizards; however, these vessels are not commonly used for several reasons. The cephalic vein is usually extremely small and, because this is a blind stick, a surgical cut down is likely necessary. The ventral abdominal vein is not generally used (especially in awake animals), due to the inability to both properly restrain the animal and control hemorrhage.

Lastly, the jugular vein is not commonly used because in many species it is also a blind stick and may also require a surgical cut down to access the vessel. Lymphatic fluid contamination is also common when sampling from the jugular vein. Lymphatic fluid contamination can skew some blood values.

The most common vessel used for lizard venipuncture is the caudal tail vein, also called the ventral coccygeal vein. There are two different techniques commonly used to obtain blood from this vessel. These techniques include the lateral and ventral approach. To successfully obtain a blood sample from either approach, a 1–1.5 inch, 27- to 20-gauge needle attached to a 1 or 3 cc syringe should generally be used. The size of the needle and syringe will depend on the size lizard you are drawing blood from. Insulin syringes can be used on very small lizards, but the needle should be cut off before putting the blood into the appropriate tubes. The small needle size can cause lysis of the blood cells if pushed through the needle (the same is true for 27- or 25-gauge needles). It is important that the tail is gently restrained during the blood draw. The left hand can be used to restrain the caudal portion of the tail, while the right hand can be used to perform the blood draw. If you are left-handed, obtain your blood sample from the other side of the tail using your left hand to draw blood and your right hand to gently restrain the tail.

For a lateral approach, the needle should be inserted into the tail (between two scales) at approximately a 90° angle. The needle should be slowly inserted into the tail, keeping slight negative pressure on the syringe until either blood enters the syringe or the needle touches the vertebrae. If the needle touches the vertebrae, slowly back it off the bone (still keeping slight negative pressure on the syringe) and redirect the needle into the vessel. It is important to put only slight negative pressure on the syringe while obtaining the blood sample. Too much negative pressure may collapse the vessel.

The technique for the ventral midline approach is very similar to the lateral approach. The needle should be inserted on midline into the tail (between two scales) at approximately a 90° angle. The needle should be slowly inserted into the tail, keeping slight negative pressure on the syringe until either blood enters the syringe or the needle touches the vertebrae. The blood vessel is located just ventral to the vertebrae. If the vertebrae is touched first, slowly back off of the bone until your needle is seated within the vessel.

Lizards usually struggle when they are placed on their backs, making it difficult to obtain a sample. The authors prefer to keep animals in sternal recumbence while obtaining the blood sample.

Chelonians

The brachial plexus, subcarapacial venous sinus, and jugular vein are the major sites where blood is collected in chelonians. The venipuncture site will depend on the size and species of the patient and the preference of the phlebotomist. If drawing blood from the jugular vein, the turtle or tortoise should be placed in lateral recumbency. The head and neck should be pulled away from the shell. The jugular vein can be found in the same plane as the eye and the tympanum. To obtain the sample, the phlebotomist will hold the head while the restrainer restrains the patient in lateral recumbency. The restrainer will usually occlude the vessel for the phlebotomist using either a finger or cotton tipped applicator. A 27- to 20-gauge needle attached to a 1 or 3 cc syringe is generally used and will vary depending on the size of the patient (Figure 13.8).

The subcarapacial venous sinus is often used when jugular venipuncture is not an option (Figure 13.9). Depending on the size of the patient, a 1–1.5 inch

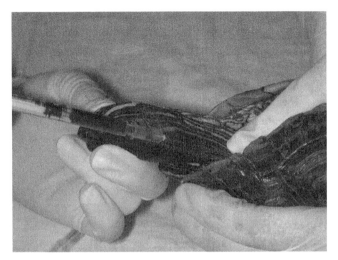

Figure 13.8 Collecting blood via the jugular vein in chelonians.

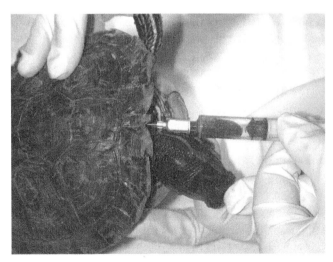

Figure 13.9 Using the subcarapacial venous sinus when the jugular venipuncture is not an option.

27- to 20-gauge needle or a 2 inch spinal needle attached to a 1 or 3 cc syringe is used to obtain the blood sample. The needle is inserted upward at about a 60-degree angle just dorsal to the neck. Slight negative pressure should be applied on the syringe until either blood enters the syringe or bone is encountered. If bone is encountered, the needle should be backed off the bone and redirected slightly.

The brachial plexus, also called the ulnar venous plexus, can be used in most chelonians. The front limb is first pulled away from the body so that the tendon near the radiohumeral joint can be palpated. Generally, a 22- to 20-gauge needle attached to a 1 or 3 cc syringe is inserted at a 90-degree angle to skin and angled toward the radiohumeral joint. This site works well for patients that are not allowing restraint of the head and neck. It is important to remember that this is a sinus and not a true blood vessel. Anytime a sinus is used for blood sampling, the chance for lymphatic fluid contamination is present.

The tail vein can be used for blood collection in chelonian patients. Either the dorsal or ventral aspect of the tail can be cannulated. The lateral approach is much more difficult and is rarely used in most species. The same technique used in lizards can also be applied to chelonian species. The tail often has feces and urate contamination. If the tail is used, it should be washed with soap and water prior to inserting a needle under the skin.

Snakes

The two primary venipuncture sites in snakes include the caudal tail vein and the heart. Drawing blood from the tail vein is best accomplished in larger snakes, due to the size of the vessel. The same method used to draw blood from the ventral midline approach in lizards is used in snakes as well. Drawing blood using a lateral approach is possible, but the shape of the vertebrae in snakes makes it much more difficult.

Obtaining a blood sample from the heart (also called cardiocentesis) is generally the quickest method that will yield the largest amount of blood. A 27- to 22-gauge needle attached to a 1 or 3 cc syringe is used for blood collection (size of needles and syringes will depend on the size of the snake). To obtain a blood sample, the snake should first be placed into dorsal recumbency. The heart is located in the cranial third of the body. The heart can move both cranially and caudally; therefore it is best to place the thumb and index finger on either side of the heart to stabilize the positioning. Prior to insertion of the needle, it is important to look for the caudal portion of the beating heart. The needle insertion site is two scutes (scales) below that. To collect blood, the needle should be inserted between two scutes at a 45-degree angle. It is important to not poke around searching for the heart. The needle should be inserted in one fluid motion and seated into the ventricle. Slight negative pressure should be placed on the syringe so that the beating of the heart slowly fills the syringe. See Figure 13.10.

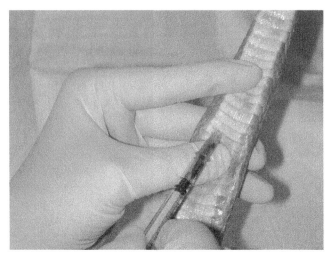

Figure 13.10 Cardiocentesis is commonly used for blood collection in the snake.

The palatine vessels can be used in some instances, but this technique is not suggested, as it is difficult to provide hemostasis, the vessels are very small, and the mouth is filled with bacteria.

Clipping a toenail to obtain a blood sample is sometimes suggested when other sites are not easily assessable. There are many negative issues with this technique. In the authors' opinion, this technique is painful and unethical. This technique would not be practiced on a dog or cat and human physicians would never do this; therefore we should follow suite with exotic species. The feet are also very dirty. Reptiles walk through feces and urates. Even when the feet are cleaned, there is still a chance for contamination. Lastly, infection can be introduced into a nail that was cut too short. Chemical restraint should be considered when samples cannot be obtained via traditional methods.

Obtaining arterial samples in reptiles is rarely done in a clinical setting. The most common artery used for sample collection is the carotid artery. A surgical cut-down must be performed to gain access to this vessel.

Amphibians

Respiratory system

Amphibian gas exchange occurs via multiple different modes. Larval stage amphibians and neotenic species (adults that retain larval traits) rely on gills. Adult amphibians have a similar lung structure and physiology to reptiles in that they are sac-like. However, pulmonic respiration depends on axial and appendicular muscle of a species. Adult amphibian species can also have significant gas exchange via cutaneous and buccopharyngeal means. Cutaneous respiration is less efficient, and buccopharyngeal respiration is highly dependent on the pumping action of the larynx, the throat movement commonly seen in frog or toad species. It is important to note the tissue must be moist for cutaneous or buccopharyngeal respiration to occur (Campbell 2004c; Helmer & Whiteside 2005c).

Renal function and osmoregulation

The body mass of amphibians is 75–80% water. Amphibians have mesonephric kidneys and are unable to concentrate urine above the solute concentrations of their plasma. Urine enters a bi-lobed bladder from excretion into the cloaca. Excretion of nitrogenous wastes depends on habitat and the need to conserve water. Larva and most adults excrete ammonia through kidneys, gills, and skin. Terrestrial species convert toxic ammonia into less toxic urea via the liver, then stored in the bladder until the animal can spare water to release through urination. Certain species conserve even more water by converting nitrogen wastes into uric acid, while others convert ammonia to urea based on water availability (Campbell 2004c; Helmer & Whiteside 2005c).

Electrolyte and acid-base

Electrolyte regulation in amphibians is highly variable. Dietary uptake is certainly part of the normal physiology, but so is transepithelial absorption from surrounding water of sodium and chloride. Transepithelial means of electrolyte accumulation is dependent on urea in the blood to assist with ion transfer. Sodium and chloride levels are generally about 10 times great than potassium levels (Duellman & Trueb 1986). Amphibians are particularly interesting when it comes to acid-base regulation. We still know very little when it comes to their regulatory mechanisms of any of their systems, in particular their acid-base systems. Amphibians have an added layer of complexity to this homeostatic regulatory system with transepithelial ion exchange. Most of the acid-base studies thus far have only investigated their air sacs under ventilator control. Until relatively recently a strong thermal dependence of ion concentrations relating to air-breathing amphibians acid-base was missing. The cane toad was the model used to show large reductions in plasma electrolyte concentrations with drops in thermal gradients, which then significantly changes the hydration status of the animal. It is speculated the water retention was due to the change of set point for osmoregulation and reduced kidney function. The study also showed that the once common belief of air-breathing amphibians using respiratory and physiochemical changes to adjust pH in varying temperature gradients was false (Feder 1992; Stinner and Hartzler 2000).

Collection sites

Collection sites in most amphibious patients include the lingual venous plexus, femoral vein, and ventral abdominal vein. The ventral abdominal vein is most commonly used across multiple species. An insulin syringe or 1 cc syringe with a 27-gauge needle attached is most commonly used for sample collection.

Fish

Respiratory system

Living fully submerged in water where there is less oxygen and it is more difficult to extract provides challenges to the adaptation and physiology of aquatic animal respiratory systems. Fish have evolved a very efficient respiratory mechanism for extracting oxygen in water in the form of gills. Gills are, however, susceptible to parasites and because of their exposure to water can suffer damage from poor water quality or chemicals. Unlike mammals, fish ventilation is unidirectional and not bidirectional. Water will fill the buccal cavity, and then close, thereby opening the opercula and pushing the water over the gills. This is called the dual phase pump method. Some fish species will more commonly swim with their mouth open, thus alleviating the energy requirement for the dual-phase pump method, while others will only use this method when encountering a counter current. Fish can cough to expel debris or after gill irritation, moving water in the reverse of normal flow. Depending on the gill size to fish ratio one can determine the fish's activity level or tolerance to hypoxia. Fish with larger sets of gills are generally more active or live in less oxygenated water.

Gills not only help oxygenate the fish but also serves in osmoregulation, excretion of nitrogenous waste, and acid-base regulation. The basic anatomy of most boney fish (teleosts) comprises four gill arches on each side, one non-respiratory pseudobranch on each side, two opercula, and the buccal cavity.

The gill arches have two distinct rows of gill filaments, giving a comb-like appearance. Less visible to the naked eye are the secondary filaments on the primary filaments to increase. These secondary filaments are covered in only 1–2 layers of micro-ridged epithelial cells to increase surface area with a core vascular space where gas exchange occurs. Like avian and reptilian species, the respiratory capillaries are so small erythrocytes must enter single file in and out of the vascular space. Finally, the gills are covered in a biofilm of mucus and other components for protection. The most superficial layers of epithelium are sensitive to environmental changes and the stress of the fish. Fish can undergo catecholamine-mediated reactions from stress which will increase blood flow to the gills for increased oxygen uptake.

Certain species of fish (catfish, bettas, gouramis, paradise fish, and labyrinth fish) have evolved highly vascularized accessory organs that allows for "air breathing." This adaptation is especially useful in environments where water can become depleted of oxygen or if the fish must bury themselves in mud during dry seasons (Roberts & Smith 2011).

Renal function

Freshwater boney fish have kidneys with well-developed glomeruli, proximal and distal tubules, and collecting ducts, while lacking a loop of Henle. The proximal tubules are divided into two units, which is unique to fish. Freshwater fish maintain a high glomerular filtration rate and urine production, due to sodium loss and constant water loading. Sodium chloride is reabsorbed in the renal tubules and collection ducts. Ion reabsorption is considerable in their water-permeable "urinary bladder." Fish lack a true urinary bladder, but instead have an enlarged distal ureter that resemble a bladder made of mesothelial cells.

Saltwater fish have significantly less and smaller glomeruli compared to their freshwater cousins, while lacking a loop of Henle. They may even lack a distal tubule. In some species glomeruli and proximal tubules may also be missing in some species. Just the opposite of freshwater fish, marine fish are under constant threat of water depletion and salt loading. Reabsorption of necessary solutes occurs in the water permeable "urinary bladder" (Campbell 2004c).

Electrolyte and acid-base

Fish gills have mitochondria-rich cells where it is postulated that a majority of ionic and acid-base regulation occurs of certain solutes. Both freshwater and marine fish have evolved osmotic and ionic regulatory mechanisms, allowing for a semi-constant plasma and intracellular sodium level. The same is true with cellular volume. Potassium regulation is similar to reptiles, and while calcium is readily available in fresh and saltwater, fish must limit their intake.

Acid-base regulation is highly variable among fish, due to the rapid changes in water temperature, electrolyte composition, oxygenation, and CO_2 levels. Because the gills are a major site for gas exchange and ion regulation, fluctuations are constant. Compared to land animals, fish have relatively low CO_2 concentrations. Respiration has little regulatory effect on acid-base in fish. Fish are capable of ionic transfer for acid-base regulation to some extent across the skin and kidney (Campbell 2004c; Ballentyne 2014).

Collection sites

Fish are most commonly anesthetized for any procedure including physical examination and blood collection (Figure 13.11). Venous and arterial blood is obtained via the caudal tail vein and artery respectively. Total circulating blood volume in fish is approximately 5%. Because the hemodynamics of fish is different from that of mammals, approximately 30–50% of blood can be collected for sampling, although this volume is rarely needed. A 1 cc syringe with a 27- or 25-gauge needle attached is generally used for sampling (Figure 13.12).

Conclusion

Blood gas analysis and evaluation of electrolyte imbalances can be challenging in exotic animal patients. Due to the lack of published data, even in the most commonly kept fish, amphibians, reptiles, birds, and exotic small mammals, veterinary professionals are often forced to extrapolate from domestic species. While this is generally helpful, much more research is needed in this area of medicine.

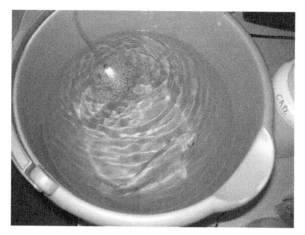

Figure 13.11 Fish are anesthetized for basic physical examinations and diagnostic procedures including blood collection. The most common anesthetic used is tricaine methanesulfonate (MS-222).

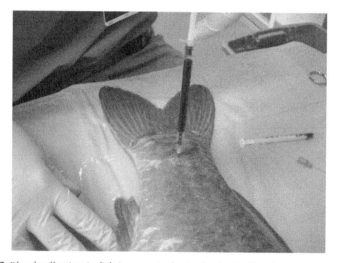

Figure 13.12 Blood collection in fish is very similar to that in the lizard.

For those working with or wanting to work with exotic animals, it is important to stay current on scientific literature and attend advanced continuing education as this field continues to develop and expand.

References

Ballentyne, J. (2014). Membranes and metabolism. In: D. Evens, J. Claiborne, & S. Currie (eds), *The Physiology of Fishes*, 4th ed. Boca Raton, FL: CRC Press: 112–115.

Boggs, D., Kilgore, D., & Birchard, G. (1984). Respiratory physiology of burrowing mammals and birds. *Comparative Biochemistry and Physiology* **77**a: 1–7.

Bounous, D. I. (2010). Avian and reptile hematology. In: B. Ballard & R. Cheek (eds), *Exotic Animal Medicine for the Veterinary Technician*, 2nd ed. Ames, IA: Wiley-Blackwell: 387–93.

Bradshaw, S., Morris, K., & Bradshaw, F. (2001). Water and electrolyte homeostasis and kidney function of desert-dwelling marsupial wallabies in Western Australia. *Journal of Comparative Physiology* **171**(1): 22–32.

Campbell, T. (2004a). Clinical chemistry of birds. In: M. Thrall, D. Baker, T. Campbell, et al. (eds), *Veterinary Hematology and Clinical Chemistry*. Baltimore: Lippincott Williams & Wilkins: 479–85.

Campbell, T. (2004b). Clinical chemistry of reptiles. In: M. Thrall, D. Baker, T. Campbell, et al. (eds), *Veterinary Hematology and Clinical Chemistry*. Baltimore: Lippincott Williams & Wilkins: 493–8.

Campbell, T. (2004c). Clinical chemistry of fish and amphibians. In: M. Thrall, D. Baker, T. Campbell, et al. (eds), *Veterinary Hematology and Clinical Chemistry*. Baltimore: Lippincott Williams & Wilkins: 499–501.

Carpenter. J. W. (2013). *Exotic Animal Formulary*. St Louis, MO: Elsevier Saunders.

Davenport, J. (1992). Sleep, torpor and hibernation. In: *Animal Life at Low Temperature*. London: Chapman & Hall: 124–7.

Carpenter, J. W., Klaphake, E., & Gibbons, P. M. (2014). Reptile formulary and normal values. In: D. R. Mader & S. J. Divers (eds), *Current Therapy in Reptile Medicine and Surgery*. St Louis, MO: Elsevier Saunders: 382–410.

Dessauer, H. (1970). Blood chemistry of reptiles: Physiological and evolutionary aspects. In: C. Gans & T. S. Parsons (eds), *Biology of the Reptilia*. Academic Press, London: 1–47.

Duellman, W. & Trueb, L. (1986). *Biology of Amphibians*. Baltimore: JHU Press: 28.

Feder, M. (1992). *Environmental Physiology of the Amphibians*. Chicago: University of Chicago Press: 118–121.

Gibbons, P. W. (2014). Therapeutics. In: D. R. Mader & S. J. Divers, *Current Therapy in Reptile Medicine and Surgery*. St Louis, MO: Elsevier Saunders: 57–69.

Harms, C., Mallo, K., Ross, P. et al. (2003). Venous blood gases and lactates of wild loggerhead sea turtles (*Caretta caretta*) following two capture techniques. *Journal of Wildlife Diseases* **39**(2): 366–74.

Harr, K. E. (2006). Diagnostic value of biochemistry. In: G. J. Harrison & T. L. Lightfoot (eds), *Clinical Avian Medicine: Volume II*. Palm Beach, FL: Spix Publishing Inc.: 612–630.

Hartzler, L., Munns, S., Bennet, A. et al. (2006). Metabolic and blood gas dependence on digestive state in the Savannah monitor lizard *Varanus exanthematicus*: An assessment of the alkaline tide. *Journal of Experimental Biology* **209**: 1052–7.

Helmer, P. & Whiteside, D. (2005a). Avian anatomy and physiology. In: B. O'Malley (ed.), *Clinical Anatomy and Physiology of Exotic Species*. Edinburgh: Elsevier Saunders: 97–137.

Helmer, P. & Whiteside, D. (2005b). General anatomy and physiology of reptiles. In: B. O'Malley (ed.), *Clinical Anatomy and Physiology of Exotic Species*. Edinburgh: Elsevier Saunders: 17–77.

Helmer, P. & Whiteside, D. (2005c). Amphibian anatomy and physiology. In: B. O'Malley (ed.), *Clinical Anatomy and Physiology of Exotic Species*. Edinburgh: Elsevier Saunders: 9–12.

Helmer, P., Lewingtin, J., & Whiteside, D. (2005). Small mammals. In: B. O'Malley (ed.), *Clinical Anatomy and Physiology of Exotic Species*. Edinburgh: Elsevier Saunders: 165–237.

Lennox, A. M. & Bauck, L. (2012). Basic anatomy, physiology, husbandry, and clinical techniques. In: K. E. Queensberry & J. W. Carpenter (eds), *Ferrets, Rabbits, and Rodents Clinical Medicine and Surgery*, 3rd ed. St Louis, MO: Elsevier Saunders: 339–53.

Long, S. (1981). Acid-base balance and urinary acidification in birds. *Comparative Biochemistry and Physiology* **71**(4): 519–526.

Longley L. A. (ed.), (2008). Reptile anesthesia. In: *Anesthesia of Exotic Pets*. St Louis, MO: Elsevier Saunders: 185–241.

Marder J. & Arad Z. (1989). Panting and acid-base regulation in heat stressed birds. *Comparative Biochemistry and Physiology* **94**(3): 395–400.

McWhorter, T. & Del Rio, C. M. (1999). Food ingestion and water turnover in hummingbirds: How much dietary water is absorbed? *Journal of Experimental Biology* **202**: 2851–8.

Roberts, H. & Smith, S. (2011). Disorders of the respiratory system in pet and ornamental fish. In: S. Orosz & C. Johnson-Delaney (eds), *Veterinary Clinics of North America: Exotic animal practice*. Philadelphia: Elsevier Saunders: 179–81.

Schumacher, J. & Mans, C. (2014). Anesthesia. In: D. R. Mader & S. J. Divers (eds), *Current Therapy in Reptile Medicine and Surgery*. St Louis, MO: Elsevier Saunders: 134–53.

Stinner, J. & Hartzler, L. (2000). Effect of temperature on pH and electrolyte concentration in air-breathing ectotherms. *Journal of Experimental Biology* **203**: 2065–74.

West, J. (2009). Comparative physiology of the pulmonary blood-gas barrier: The unique avian solution. *American Journal of Physiology* **297**(6): 1625–34.

Index

acid-base, 1
    analysis, 117–120
acid-base disorders, 102–120
    metabolic, 107–110, 121–135
    mixed, 152–162
    respiratory, 107–113, 136–151
acid-base-traditional approach,
        102–120
acidemia, 2, 3, 122
acidity, 2
acidosis, 122
acute lung injury (ALI), 150
acute respiratory distress syndrome (ARDS),
        141, 143, 150
acute tumor lysis syndrome, 76
albumin, 169
ALI see acute lung injury (ALI)
alkalemia, 3, 122
alkalosis, 122
    chloride resistant, 167
    chloride responsive, 167
Alveolar arterial gradient, (A-a gradient),
        149–150
amphibians-chapter, 13
    electrolyte and acid-base, 201
    renal function, 201
    respiratory system, 200–201
anion, 5, 34
anion gap, 10, 115–116, 125–126,
        157–158
ARDS see acute respiratory distress
        syndrome (ARDS)
arrhythmia, 52
$A_{[TOT]}$, 169

atrial natriuretic peptide, 20
avian see birds

base excess, 116–117, 124
    approach, 171–172
bicarbonate, 54, 104–105
birds, 186–188
    acid-base, 188–189
    electrolytes, 188–189
    renal function, 187–188
    respiratory system, 186–187
Boyles law, 103
Bronsted and Lowry, 2
buffer, 3, 105–106, 123–124

calcium, 79–101
    regulation, 79–85
calcium gluconate, 53
calcium oxalate crystals, 132
capnography, 125, 178
carbon dioxide, 104, 124–125, 139, 170
carbonic acid, 2, 124–125
cation, 5
cerebral edema, 23
chloride, 5, 34–43
    chloride gap, 37
    homeostasis, 35
    sodium to chloride difference, 38
    sodium:chloride ratio, 36, 38
chloride resistant metabolic alkalosis, 129
chloride responsive metabolic alkalosis, 129
compensation, strong ion, 171
compensatory response, 127–128
congestive heart failure, 25

diabetes insipidus, 38
diabetes mellitus, 22
diabetic ketoacidosis, 39, 126, 132
diffusion impairment, 149

eclampsia, 87–88
electrolytes, 4
end tidal CO_2 ($ETCO_2$), 178–179
ethylene glycol, 126, 133
exotics, 175–206
  catheterization, 177
  pH, 177–178
  renal function, 180–181
  respiratory system, 179–180
  sample collection, 175–176,
      181—186
    amphibians, 201
    avian, 189–190
    chelonians, 197–199
    chinchillas, 182
    ferrets, 181—182
    fish, 203
    guinea pigs, 183–185
    lizard, 196–197
    rabbits, 182–183
    rodents, 185–186
    snakes, 199–200
  sample storage, 176

factitious hyponatremia *see* normo-osmolar
      hyponatremia
fish, 202
  electrolyte and acid-base, 203
  renal function, 202–203
  respiratory system, 202
fraction of inspired oxygen, (FiO_2),
      143–144
free water deficit, 32

heatstroke, 132
Henderson–Hasselbalch, 102–103
  equation, 122
hibernation, 180
hydrogen, 122–123
hydrogen Ions, 2
hyperadrenocorticism, 38, 41, 48
hyperaldosteronism, 29, 41, 60, 71, 73,
      129, 168
hypercalcemia, 92–98
hypercapnia, 141

hyperchloremia, 38–40
  artifactual, 38
  corrected, 39
  iatrogenic, 40
  psuedochyperchloremia, 38
hyperglycemic-hyperosmolar non-ketotic
      syndrome (HHNS), 22
hyperkalemia, 50–54
  causes, 50–51
  treatment, 53–54
hyperlipdemia, 21
hypermagnesemia, 63–64
  causes, 63
  treatment, 64
hypernatremia, 28–33
hyperosmolality, 22–24
  hypervolemic, 29
  hypovolemic, 29
  normovolemic, 29
hyperosmolar hyponatremia, 22,
      27, 30
hyperparathyroidism, 98–99
hyperphosphatemia, 75–76
  causes, 76–77
hyperproteinemia, 21
hypoadrenocorticism, 25, 63
hypocalcemia, 86–91
hypochloremia, 40–42
  artifactual, 41
  chloride resistant, 41
  corrected, 41
hypochloremic alkalosis, 37
hypokalemia, 47–50, 129–130
  causes of, 48
  treatment, 49
hypomagnesemia, 59–62
  causes, 59–60
  treatment, 61–62
hyponoatremia, 20, 28
  hyperosmolar, 22–24
  hypervolemic, 25–26
  hypoosmolar, 24–28
  hypovolemic, 24–25
  normoosmolar, 21
  normovolemic, 26
hypoparathyroidism, 77
hypophosphatemia, 70–75
  causes, 70–73
  treatment, 74–75
hypotonic fluid loss, 38

hypoventilation, 148
hypoxic, 141

idiogenic osmoles, 23, 30
insulin, 53
intranasal cannula, 148

Kussmaul respiration, 40, 122

lactic acid, 131–132
liver failure, 25
loop diuretics, 129

magnesium, 57–65
  regulation, 58–59
metabolic, 3, 110–114
    acidosis, 55, 114, 131–134
    alkalosis, 38, 49, 114, 128–131
    prognosis, 134
mixed acid-base disorders, 126–127,
        152–162
    chloride, 158
    compensation, 153–154
    effects of, 159
    evaluating, 158–159
    metabolic, 156
    respiratory, 153–155
    treatment, 161
Myxedema coma, 26

nasal prongs, 145–148
natriuresis, 26, 31
nephrotic syndrome, 25
non-volatile buffer acidosis, 170
non-volatile buffer alkalosis,
        169–170
normo-osmolar hyponatremia, 21

osmolality, 14–15, 21
osmoles, 7–9
osmolytes *see* idiogenic osmoles
osmoreceptors, 17
osmotic demyelination syndroms
        (ODS), 27
osmotic diuresis, 32, 38, 40
oxygen, 138–139
oxygenation, 137–138
oxygen cage, 148
    hemoglobin disassociation curve, 139
    hood, 146, 148

therapy, 148
supplementation, 148

PaO_2:FiO_2, 150
partial pressure of arterial carbon
        dioxide($PaCO_2$), 139–141
partial pressure of arterial
        oxygen(PaO_2), 138
pH, 2, 104, 121–123
phosphorus, 66–78
    regulation, 67–68
point-of-care device, 130
potassium, 5, 44–56
    regulation, 44–45
potassium gluconate, 49
power of hydrogen, 122
primary acid-base disturbance, 126
primary hypodipsia, 29
pseudohyperkalemia, 52–53
pseudohyponatremia *see* normo-osmolar
        hyponatremia
psychogenic polydipsia, 26

renal, 3
    failure, 88–89
    tubular acidosis, 39
renin-angiotensin aldosterone system,
        18–19
reptiles, 191–200
    acid-base, 193–196
    electrolytes, 193–196
    renal function, 192–193
    respiratory system, 191–192
respiratory, 3, 107–110, 136–151
    acidosis, 109, 139–142
    alkalosis, 110, 142–143
right to left shunt, 150

sampling errors, 161–162
secondary acid-base disturbance, 126
shock, 131–132
SIADH *see* syndrome of inappropriate
        anti-diuretic hormone
        (SIADH)
simple acid-base disorders, 126–127
simplified strong ion model, 172
sodium, 5, 13–32
    corrected sodium calculation, 22
    distribution, 14–15
    reabsorption, 16

sodium (*cont'd*)
  regulation, 16–17
  and water balance, 13, 32
sodium bicarbonate, 133–134
sodium/potassium pump, 45–47
Sorenson, 2
Stewart, 103
Stewart-Figge Method, 171
strong ion gap, 172–173
Syndrome of inappropriate anti-diuretic
    hormone (SIADH), 26

temperature, 126
thirst response, 17
translocational hyponatremia *see*
    hyperosmolar hyponatremia

urine chloride, 128

vasopressin, 17
V/Q mismatch, 149

water deficit, free, 29